A Piece of My Mind

Edited by Roxanne K. Young

A New Collection of Essays From JAMA

The Journal of the American Medical Association

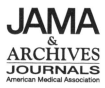

JAMA
&
ARCHIVES
JOURNALS
American Medical Association

AMA Press

Vice President: Anthony J. Frankos

Editorial Director: Mary Lou White

Managing Editor: Patricia Dragisic

Senior Editor: Robin Husayko

Production and Manufacturing: Jean Roberts (Director)
Rosalyn Carlton
Anne Serrano
Ronnie Summers

Sales and Marketing: Mike Desposito (Director)
J.D. Kinney
Patrick Dati

JAMA **Book Liaison:** Annette Flanagin

Additional copies may be ordered from:
Order Department OP031700
ISBN 1-57947-082-3

American Medical Association
For order information, call toll-free 800-621-8335
BA62:04-P-045: 9/04

An excerpt of the poem "Talking to the Family" was reprinted with permission from
The Smell of Matches by John Stone. Originally published by Rutgers University Press, 1972.
Reprinted by LSU Press, 1988. Copyright 1972 by John Stone.

The quotation on page xvii of the Introduction was taken from "Sudden Intimacies"
by Michael Radetsky, MD, from the first volume of *A Piece of My Mind*.

The poem "Suzanne" by William Carlos Williams, from *Collected Poems 1939-1962*, volume II, copyright
1948 by William Carlos Williams. Reprinted by permission of New Directions Publishing Corporation.

To the physicians, nurses, patients,
and their families whose true-life stories
form the basis for these essays.

Table of Contents

The "Practice" of Medicine

All in the Family

The Dark Side

Thanks for the Memories

The View From Here

Acknowledgment

Thanks and appreciation to George D. Lundberg, MD, and Catherine D. DeAngelis, MD, former and current editors of *JAMA*; and to M. Therese Southgate, MD, Senior Contributing Editor, *JAMA*, legendary fine-art specialist, mentor, and friend.

For providing reviews, advice, feedback, support, and encouragement: to all of the other *JAMA* editors, past and present; singled out: Annette Flanagin, RN, MA, Managing Senior Editor; Juliana Walker, Assistant Editor; and Phil B. Fontanarosa, MD, Executive Deputy Editor.

Special thanks to Patricia Dragisic and Robin Husayko, AMA Press editors, for editorial support; and to Lenette Gardner, Fanny Brown, and Celina Canchola for technical support.

And, on a more personal level, to my parents, Frank and Carolyn, and my husband, Norris. And to my late brother, Charles.

Foreword

Although the practice of medicine is suffused with narrative, the stories in this collection represent a kind that is seldom heard and often left untold. Still, over the last 20 years, nearly a thousand of them have appeared in *JAMA*'s regular section "A Piece of My Mind." Now widely imitated in other medical and public health journals, these insiders' accounts of medical practice constitute a secret history of what it has been like to take care of the ill (or in some stories to *be* ill) at the end of the 20th century.

Medical attention begins with the physician's listening to the patient's account of illness. Interpreting that story and constructing from it a medical account of disease is the fundamental clinical act. The physician matches the patient's story to a taxonomy of roughly similar stories, refines it with questions and (frequently) with test results, and then translates it into a medical narrative: a recognizable disease whose plot (both physician and patient hope) can be altered therapeutically. Physicians think using such narratives, and clinical education at every level teaches and reinforces this interpretive narrative process. Although patients would be hard pressed to recognize their stories once they have been thus translated, this interpretation (and the diagnostic recognition) is part of what they have come to the doctor for.

But what happens to the terror, the life interrupted, the uneasiness, even the pain? Because these feelings and personal experiences do not promote the identification of disease, there is no place for them in the medical case. After diagnosis and treatment, what happens next? Insofar as the answer belongs to the patient's world, it is omitted from the clinical narrative. Patients' stories are not the only ones excluded. Accounts of physicians' experiences are not just irrelevant but unthinkable in the medical case. The reason for the prohibition is a sound one: a physician's personal response to the patient and the patient's illness seems to violate the ideal of an objective, standardized, replicable view of the case. Because the goal is an accurate diagnosis and choice of treatment that would be the same no matter who the physician might be, reports of a physician's experience of caring for the patient are entirely out of place in the medical report. There's all that suspect emotion!

Physicians, of course, are not made of steel. Increasingly it has been argued that medical practice is more rewarding, perhaps actually qualitatively better, if the doctor understands and appreciates his or her part in the patient-physician relationship. Doctors need a "safe" way of being in intimate contact with the horrors—and wonders—of human life. This is a need that the ideal of scientific objectivity promises to fill but seldom delivers without penalty.

Physicians have their own stories to tell. Just as patients have been telling their stories in ever-growing numbers in recent years, so also have physicians begun to tell about the emotional work of taking care of patients and the meaning of being a physician. As described in "Haying": "I feel heavy after a day's work, as if all my patients were inside me, letting me carry them. I don't mean to. But where do I put their stories?"

Here they are in abundance.

This is the second collection of *JAMA*'s "Pieces." The first, published in 1988, was arranged from birth to death. This one begins with the start of clinical education—one student jamming the pockets of a white coat the night before the first day in the hospital; another medical student working with a cadaver in gross anatomy class and imagining the life of the person who died. And it ends with (maybe the best told of all) the close of a lifetime of practice: a physician still teaching, perhaps most effectively now, as a younger physician's desperately ill patient. Most of these "Pieces" are by physicians and medical students; a few are by nurses, social workers, patients, or family members. The authors are not the "boys in white," challenging the world and conquering disease. They are men and women taking care of patients and their families, thinking and feeling at all hours, conquering fear, getting past aversion, and discovering the meaning of their profession. They tell about the little ironies, the sad times, the good ones, especially the good moments that unexpectedly emerge from bad ones. Sometimes they discover their roles have doubled, suddenly conflicting: second-generation physicians burying their physician fathers and their small-town single practices; others who suddenly, unexpectedly, are patients themselves or, worse, are the loved ones of the seriously ill or dying.

Here is the evidence that despite everything, despite the cadavers and the sleeplessness, the long hours and the exposure to death and human misery, the exhaustion and impatience with human need in the middle of the night, being a doctor doesn't make a person different in the ways that really count. We hear about the unexpectedly restorative encounters after what till then had seemed an endless day; the heartbreaking comedy of a Monday morning HIV clinic; sustaining relationships with people who defy epidemiologic predictions for alcoholism, cholesterolemia, melanoma; the anxieties of opening a new clinic, working as a medical examiner, making house calls. Patients offer the occasions for life's lessons; occasionally they are the teachers. Some seem to embody whole chunks of recent history; others offer a bridge to experience otherwise inaccessible for reasons of class or race. We meet a homeless man, mentally ill, who can recite a sonnet by Shakespeare and a demented jazz trombonist, who, when asked to write a sentence on his mini-mental status exam, responds by writing out a measure of music. We get glimpses of other health care professions: the orderly who listens to a patient talk about dying of cancer while his family pretends he has only a virus; the LPN who takes poems along on his middle-of-the-night pill-pushing rounds. The stories are stoic, emotional, laden with ritual, told with frequent wit in medical language (there's a glossary of medical terms). Above all, they are about suffering and empathy, and the recognition that at its best, empathy is never more than approximate.

A century ago Sir William Osler counseled young physicians to adopt an attitude of detachment: aequanimitas. Rules III and IV in Samuel Shem's *The House of God* offer a more contemporary version: "At a cardiac arrest, the first procedure is to take your own pulse" and "The patient is the one with the disease." But neither sage nor satirist forbade feeling or observing the human condition carefully. It's just that, at least this time, it's not *your* condition.

Or is it? Physician-poet John Stone perfectly captured the wonder and horror of a physician's forced witness to life's difficulties in "Talking to the Family":

> They will put it together
> and take it apart.
> Their voices will buzz:
> The cut ends of their nerves
> will curl.

> I will take off the coat,
> drive home,
> and replace the light bulb in the hall.

These "Pieces," like Stone's poem, are about the moments that survive the trip home, the enforced distance, the suppression of emotion. They are about the many reasons physicians are devoted to their work. They give us not just the wisdom that accrues to the experienced physician but accounts of how hard and painful it can be to acquire that wisdom. Together they offer the hidden curriculum of clinical practice: the ways people meet death, the uses of a physician's emotion, the ways of surviving, the rewards of a life in medicine.

Kathryn Montgomery, PhD
Ethics and Human Values Program
Northwestern University Medical School
Chicago, Illinois

Introduction

Twenty years have passed since the inauguration of the "A Piece of My Mind" column in *The Journal of the American Medical Association (JAMA)*. When I was asked—as an assistant editor in 1984—by former *JAMA* editor George D. Lundberg, MD, if I wished to assume responsibility for the already-popular feature, I was both terrified and elated but—appreciating the unique opportunity—enthusiastically accepted. Two conditions were proposed to start in my term as editor: that manuscripts undergo peer review and that positively reviewed manuscripts deemed worthy for publication be presented for discussion at *JAMA*'s regular editorial meetings. As the new nonphysician content editor, I was happy to agree: peer review and my colleagues' advice have been instrumental in honing the essays—weeding out potential problems with clinical details, for example—to their present state of accuracy and appropriateness. (Readers should note, however, that over the years some treatments described in the essays may have changed or become outdated.) Most published essays have undergone the dread editorial red pen, but we strive as much as possible to retain the author's unique writing style and voice because, after all, the story belongs first to its creator.

Since 1980, more than 8,000 manuscripts have been submitted and reviewed for "A Piece of My Mind." Most of the 800 or so that were ultimately published in *JAMA* were written by practicing physicians (and their family members), but scores were also sent in by medical students, nurses and other allied health personnel, the occasional medical school dean, nonmedical professionals with an interest in medicine (such as lawyers and basic-science researchers), and, of course, patients.

Not surprisingly, during the column's early years, most of the physician-authors were men, but recently, authorship seems equally distributed between the sexes—and most likely among ethnic groups, no doubt reflecting the current demographics of medical school admissions. They represent every conceivable medical specialty, and every medical walk of life.

Why do they do it? Why do these physicians write their stories? Why do they bare their souls and open their hearts, exposing themselves to *JAMA*'s readership—to 350,000 of their peers?

Over the years I've come to realize that many have recognized "A Piece of My Mind" as a vehicle, a means by which, after having put pen to paper, they are allowed to express something that changed their lives.

What compels busy physicians to risk such close scrutiny?

I believe the simple act of writing is a catharsis. In "Tears," for example, an intern is charged with drawing blood gas levels in a 3-year-old dying of kidney disease. She was "convinced this torture was unnecessary. Danny was a no code." Worse, she cried about having to subject her young patient to what she believed was a futile, useless (and painful) procedure; her supervisors reacted to her tears as a sign of weakness, pointing out that she was "ill-equipped to be a physician." Years later, reflecting on the experience, she realizes that her patients "judge me less harshly than my professors used to. Rather than assuming my tears are signs of weakness, my patients tend to see them as my way of acknowledging that we share the vicissitudes of the human condition and that they are not alone in their sorrow." In a dramatic and metaphoric statement (and with a nod to physician-poet William Carlos Williams), she concludes that "I rarely have to pound the window with both fists now."

Writing also helps us confront troubling issues—such as guilt or fear of failure—and resolve them from within. In "A Father's Eyes," an intern—who at first appears callously disdainful through his cynical assessment of an infant's grim condition—undergoes an apparent epiphany when observing the infant's young father, who, in stunned disbelief at his son's rapid and catastrophic decline, murmurs, "I don't understand." The intern realizes his own grief—and shame at his attitude—but ultimately cannot confront either the shame or the father—and simply slips away. Yet, he wrote the story, and it stands in testament to these seemingly contradictory actions and reactions.

Sometimes, authors need to examine and to vent their frustrations with what medicine seems to have become. They yearn for "the earlier days," for simpler, yet realistically unattainable times, before our technology-driven society seemed to undermine the crucial patient-physician relationship. In "Dying to Live," a physician explains to his patient—and the patient's wife—the futility of treatment for the patient's lung and central nervous system cancer, uncontrolled diabetes, severe emphysema, coronary artery disease, and hypertension; the physician advises the husband to go home and spend some time with his loved ones. The patient instead undergoes an extensive workup at a renowned clinic, where heroic measures are proposed although the staff there agrees that the patient's condition is terminal. The patient subsequently dies in the emergency department. And the patient's wife comforts the physician.

Because many stories have to do with death, my colleagues used to tease me. "So much of what you publish is depressing," they'd admonish. But it's been said death is perhaps the most intimate moment in a person's life. In the extraordinarily moving "Taps," a young mother, who had previously lost two children at or immediately after birth, is about to deliver her third child. The time is post–World War II; the scene, a hospital that also serves a naval base. The mother's dream ("She desperately wanted a child."), however, is not to be realized—her baby is born with a rare and fatal disease and dies within moments of birth. At that most intimate moment, the "mournful strains of *Taps*," coming from the nearby base, is heard. The author, who is the mother's incredulous anesthesiologist, kisses the woman's forehead and gently eases her into sleep, "postponing for her all too briefly one of the real tragedies of life."

Often, physician-writers want simply to acknowledge and honor their patients by telling their stories. They want to thank them for helping them come to grips not only with death but with life. In "My Heroes," the author's patient—hospitalized with full-blown AIDS and all its horrific manifestations—was not to have an easy death. For the author, even more difficult to watch was the patient's 10-year-old son, who bravely visited his mom at the hospital every day. Later, at the conclusion of his mother's funeral, the child throws his arms around the author and proclaims, "Thank you, Dr Nina, for taking care of my mommy." This episode made the author realize just why she does the work she does. And how—by witnessing her patients' courage—they have helped her become a better physician.

Perhaps one of the most important reasons physicians write about their experiences is that they want to remind themselves, and others, why they entered the medical profession in the first place. The joy of being a physician. The simple human act of helping another person.

Our physician-authors have confided in us, have entrusted us with some of their most personal moments, those "sudden intimacies . . . when the human barrier cracks open to reveal what is most secret and inarticulate."

And for this we are grateful.

On *JAMA*'s pages and on those that follow, I offer you a piece—or, more precisely, 100 pieces—of my heart.

Roxanne K. Young
Chicago, Illinois
July 2000

The "Practice" of Medicine

Physicians spend their entire professional lives "practicing" their art: from premed studies of anatomy, biology, chemistry, physiology, and other non-clinical disciplines (including the more recent—and welcome—addition of the humanities) to their first encounter with a cadaver ("The Gift"). Many of the most profound—and memorable—encounters occur during rotations through the impressionable clinical years of medical school ("The Chief Complaint," "Secondary Survey," "Mrs Rodell") on through internship, residency, and fellowship ("The Intern's Vein," "When to Touch," "Healing Arts," "The Legacy"). There is the exhilaration and trepidation the day before starting private practice ("Beginnings"); the life-affirming wonderment that occurs at witnessing once again the birth of a child in an obstetrician's middle years—during the middle of the night ("The Reward"); and in retirement, an oft-reluctant surrendering of the role of healer and counselor ("Identity Matters [or Does It?]"). In the following essays, it's clear that practicing medicine is a unique, intricate, and rewarding lattice of learning and relearning.

R.K.Y.

First Day

Robert E. Murphy

I was not going to be late my first day.

I laid out my white coat the night before, carefully rearranging its contents for accessibility and balance. In the left lower pocket was the "Scut Monkey Handbook" and an ECG card and ruler. In the lower right, the "Washington manual," two Vacutainer barrels, several needles, some Vacutainer tubes, my stethoscope. The upper pocket contained a penlight, a stack of index cards, and three black pens. Through my jacket's buttonhole hung a rubber tourniquet. The inside pocket stored four tongue blades, pamphlets on the physical exam and antimicrobial therapy, and a pack of peanuts. I was ready.

I got to the CCU 30 minutes before rounds and sat down at the nurses' station. The ward clerk spotted me: "You must be the new third-year student." I wondered how she could tell.

Before I could even nod my head she continued: "Okay, I'll go over this once. Routine sticks are done at 6:30 AM. Orders need to be in the night before or you do them yourself. They need to be signed by a doctor, flagged, and put in the rack. For x-rays, fill out a yellow slip, stamp it, and give it to me. ECGs and ECHOs need a red slip and be sure it's stamped too. If you do your own sticks, panel 1's go in a red tube, PT/PTTs go in a blue tube on ice, calcium goes in a green tube on ice, and blood cultures go in the yellow tubes. Be sure to get two tubes from different sites and be sure to wipe the top of the tube with Betadine, okay?"

Then what I assumed was my team walked in. Introductions were made and everyone reminisced about his or her first day on the wards. The resident's advice was "Quit now—it just gets worse."

The intern presented the first case. He talked fast, throwing out abbreviations and numbers that everyone else understood and processed. I stood on the periphery, still trying to figure out what the patient's problem was when the first question came: "This patient has a warm lower leg, his skin is erythematous and edematous, and there is a positive Homans' sign. What do you want to do?"

Twenty eyes stared at me. This wasn't like the multiple-choice questions answered during my first two years. I mumbled something about CHF and diuretics and watched them snicker and roll their eyes. An easy follow-up question went to the fourth-year: "Why are we concerned about DVTs?" But wait, I wanted to interrupt, I know the answer to that one!

And the rest of the morning was a blur. I felt more hopelessly lost with each presentation. Each intern, resident, nurse, dietician, and ward clerk took me aside to tell me how to be an "efficient" third-year student. I learned to use the computer, how to do an arterial blood gas, where to check out x-rays, medical records, and ECG files. I didn't find time for lunch.

By 4 o'clock I had indecipherable scribbles on four pages of progress notes and nine index cards and unreadable phone numbers on the palms of my hands. I ate my peanuts.

Then the resident's teaching conference—more questions. There was nowhere to hide. After I'd missed several in a row, the resident just looked at me and said, "Did you even have physiology? The lawyers are going to be licking their chops. . . ."

After conference I started working on my two progress notes for the day; I finished at 7. The nurses constantly interrupted me with more questions: What do you want to do for Mr Jones' blood pressure? Mr Smith's diarrhea? Mrs Wilson's nausea? With every question I could only answer, "I'll have to check with the intern." I felt more and more stupid as the evening wore on.

At 8 o'clock I was told to stick Mr Hunt for cardiac enzymes. I had only drawn blood on three classmates (and missed one of those). I wanted to try my hardest to look like I knew what I was doing. I palpated a nice vein in his left arm and was ready to stick him when he said, "You know, I don't think you're supposed to draw that above the IV." Even the patients knew more than I did.

As I tried to find the vein on the right side, I started to explain why we had to draw his blood every six hours. He wanted to know the difference between a heart attack and angina, what we could see with that "sonar machine," how an ECG could tell us where his heart attack was. I enjoyed explaining what we were doing, putting the complex physiology (of which

I had only a rudimentary grasp) into simple language Mr Hunt could understand.

I missed his vein three times. I apologized and said I would get the intern. "Naw," said Mr Hunt. "Give it another shot. I know you can do it."

I was touched by his confidence in me. I tried again and failed. "One more time," he said. "You'll get it this time."

And I did.

When I apologized once more and started to leave for dinner, it was almost 9 o'clock. As I said good night, he asked, "You're one of those student doctors, aren't you?" I nodded yes and confessed that he was my first patient.

"You know," he said, "nobody had sat down and said a word to me for two days. I know you're real smart and you're a mighty nice fella. You're gonna be a good doctor, I can tell."

It was a very good first day.

A Child's Pain

Michael J. Collins, MD

I was a junior medical student doing a rotation in surgery when I was called to start an IV up in Peds. Obediently I trudged up to the fourth floor. When I got there, my coat pockets bulging with various sizes and shapes of needles, the nurse brought me in to an 11-month-old baby who was lying very still in her crib.

The nurse explained that the child had suffered horrible burns in a home fire when she was just a few weeks old and had been in the hospital ever since. She had been on Peds for so long that almost everyone (except junior medical students) knew her. She had probably been around longer than most of the residents.

The baby's main problem now was that something had gone wrong with her bowels. She had undergone a number of surgeries but was still unable to take anything by mouth. Her IV had infiltrated (*"Again!"*) and she needed another one started to continue her fluids, nutrition, and antibiotics.

The nurse left me alone with the baby. I read through her chart, fascinated by all the things that had happened to her: burns over 80% of her body, liver failure, bowel necrosis, electrolyte imbalances. She had a list of surgical procedures half an inch thick.

I was starting to feel uneasy. This was *not* going to be a simple IV to start. I was sure she was going to go bananas as soon as I pulled down the side of her crib, and there would be no nurse to help me, no one to hold the child down if she began to thrash and fight. I had tried to start IVs under those circumstances before, and I didn't want to go through it again.

But I was the oldest of eight children, had been around kids my whole life, and fancied myself quite capable of charming this little one into holding still for me. I began to hum a little tune and smiled as I lowered the side of her crib. "Don't be scared, little baby. Don't be scared," I murmured soothingly. "Everything's gonna be fine."

But I needn't have worried. My little patient didn't struggle or cry. She didn't even whimper. She just lay there looking at me. There was no fear in her eyes, but there was something worse, something beyond fear. She had the eyes of an old woman—and they were filled with despair. She seemed to recognize me for what I was. She knew that I was hopelessly larger than she, hopelessly stronger, hopelessly more powerful, and that I would have my way. She could struggle, she could resist, she could cry, but none of these things would matter. I would have my way, and I would hurt her. There was nothing she could do about it. I could see all of this in those eyes.

And I saw more. I fancied that I saw a glimmer of accusation in her eyes. Or was I reading my own guilt reflected back at me? What, after all, was I doing here? Who did I think I was? I wasn't here to help her, was I? I was here to get through my surgery rotation, to learn how to start IVs, to get a good grade. That is what brought me here, here to this room, here to her side, here with sharp needles in my pocket.

She knew all this. And she knew something else too, something no child should ever know: she knew that she did not matter. She knew that her condition, her pain, her *life* were not important. How could they be important? If they were, why was a lowly medical student here to start her IV? Why wasn't the intern here? Or the resident? Or the attending? Or, damn it, why wasn't the chief of surgery here?

But she knew why. She knew she wasn't worth their while to come. She was just an 11-month-old silent lump of burned flesh who didn't rate anyone better than a junior medical student to start her IV. She accepted this. Her eyes showed no sign of bitterness, just resignation and profound despair.

I tried to tell those eyes to be reasonable. The chief of surgery can't start *every* IV in the hospital, can't change *every* dressing, can't perform *every* surgery. And besides, this was a teaching hospital, wasn't it? How else were the rest of us to learn? Didn't she realize this?

No, that's not what she realized. What she realized was that day after day, week after week, she was made to suffer. First there had been the burns, the horrible burns, and they hurt and she cried and cried but no one came to hold her. And then these big strangers came and they hurt her more, and they kept coming, and they kept hurting her, and she cried and struggled but they held her down and hurt her more, and once when she woke up she felt sick and a big stranger came and stabbed her first in the right arm and then in the left arm, and she fought him and she cried but he swore and slammed her arm back down and stabbed her again and he ripped the flesh off her legs and she cried and cried until she couldn't cry any more, but the big strangers still came.

And they came, and they came.

And they kept coming and they kept hurting her until finally, after the fifth or 50th or 500th stranger had stabbed her or cut her or slashed her or squeezed her, she stopped struggling and stopped hoping, and just lay there with huge eyes in a tortured, emaciated, ravaged little body.

I had never seen such profound despair. I never would again. My heart went out to her and my charming words choked in my throat. This was one child who would not be amused with chirping bird noises or flashing penlights.

I hesitated, my confidence shaken like it never could have been from any loud-talking, offensive, demanding adult. Again I started to speak to her gently and quietly, trying to win her confidence and trust, but then I stopped. Win her confidence and trust—*for what?* So I could turn around and abuse it by inflicting more pain?

And then I realized that I was becoming a part of it all. I was becoming one of them. Me! No, I protested, no! I'm not here to hurt her, I'm here to help her. ("Oh, really?" those eyes responded. "I thought you were here to *practice* on me.")

I was confused, disjointed. This was just a baby, just a baby. I had an IV to start. I was here to help, to heal. My heart was in the right place. I *cared* about her. I wanted her to get better and grow up and find someone to hold her and love her and care for her. That's what I wanted. I wanted her pain to stop. I wanted her to stop having that look in her eyes. I didn't want her to look at me like that. *I* wasn't the problem. The burns were the problem. I was just helping her to get over those burns. Someday she would realize that.

But what difference did it make *what* she realized or didn't realize? The only thing that mattered was that I was going to hurt her—now. I was going to have my way. She knew that. She lay so still, so quiet. I didn't want to look at her any more. With tears in my eyes I lifted her limp, withered, scarred little arm and stabbed it; and stabbed it again; and stabbed it a third time, until finally the blood flowed. She never budged and her eyes never left my face.

I wrapped a bandage around the IV site (we wouldn't want there to be any bleeding when we were done, would we?). Wearily I raised the side of her crib, turned, and left the room. That is, I *tried* to leave the room.

I have been trying ever since.

The Gift

Michael A. Grassi

> There ought to be behind the door of every happy, contented man some-
> one standing with a hammer continually reminding him with a tap that
> there are unhappy people; that however happy he may be, life will show
> him her claws sooner or later, trouble will come for him—disease,
> poverty, losses, and no one will see or hear, just as now he neither sees
> nor hears others.
>
> Anton Chekhov, *Gooseberries*

We moved to Chicago from Bayfield, Wisconsin, in 1931. Those were
tough times. No family. No job. No money. No help. Maybe it was
partly our own doing. You see, Elsie became pregnant while we were still
dating. I did not have much of a family to speak of. My mother died
when I was 5, and while my father housed and fed me and my brothers,
he did nothing more. Elsie's family was big and stable. Her father had a
job, which was something in those days. I thought her parents might
help us get a start in life, but once they heard about the baby, that was it.
Elsie and I were on our own. That was made very clear. After our wedding we left for Chicago, intent on making things work out, praying that
I could find a job to support us.

I landed a job as a butcher up in the old meatpacking district by
Fulton Street. But that is not how I started out. I began as a hauler.
Haulers were responsible for hauling the sides of beef off the trucks and
into the coolers. I worked my butt off. No one, probably to this day, can
haul a side of beef like me. It got to the point where I would carry one
on each shoulder. Eight hours a day I would work like this.

Still we couldn't make ends meet. Eating oatmeal for dinner three or
four nights a week is no way to live, especially since we now had a son.
So, I took on another job bartending at a neighborhood joint, Marty's

Tap. I would haul from 6 in the morning until 3 and then bartend usually from 4 until midnight or so. It was not meant to become a permanent arrangement, but even after I became a butcher (fastest promotion in Glascott's history), I kept on bartending for the extra money.

Our one-bedroom basement apartment gave way to a three-bedroom midrise on the North Side. By this time, Elsie was working too, at Brach's candy, and we had a baby daughter. Though things were coming together, they were never all that together. I don't care if you get married when you are 30 or at 18 like us; you are still going to have problems, and we had ours.

I was gone a lot during the week because of work. But this pattern started to include the weekends too. I started drinking with fellas from the bar, shooting stick for too much money, and catting around. It became pretty bad. Elsie and I would get into these terrible fights, after which I would just head back to the bar. Things kept on this way for awhile, Elsie and I growing further apart. I know more than half the reason we stayed together for those years was the kids, John and Angie.

For 20 years I worked those two jobs. Elsie stayed on at Brach's, and we did all right. Our kids both graduated from high school and are doing pretty well. John is in Georgia where he is a financial planner, and Angie is married, three kids now, and still lives in Chicago. I don't think Elsie and I did that bad for two tenth-grade dropouts.

Life took its toll on both of us, though. Elsie had a stroke from 40 years of smoking those stupid Pall Malls. And me, well, my liver isn't in that great of shape from those years of drinking, though I haven't had a sip in 30 years. You know why I stopped? It wasn't anything Elsie said. Rather, when Angie was 17 or so, she had a pretty serious boyfriend. They were dating for maybe six months, and I still hadn't met him. I told Angie to bring him by, but she refused. She said she didn't want me to embarrass her in front of this boy that she liked so much. Even though I only drank on the weekends and it never affected my job, I quit then. That was it.

Oddly enough, my health problems didn't stem so much from my drinking as from my eating. I would bring home steaks, pork roasts, and beef shanks almost every evening from Glascott's. Breakfast was three eggs, four pancakes, and sausage at Ruby's Diner before work. I was young and strong. Even if I had known about cholesterol, I wouldn't have cared. I am still not so sure what it is even now. But I paid for it with three heart attacks, one ending in a quadruple bypass. It was the last one that killed me. I just wasn't strong enough any more to keep fighting.

I am lying here in front of you now because of those doctors that saved me the first two times. They gave me 15 years I would never have had. Fifteen years to make things right with Elsie. To care for her after her stroke as she cared for me and the children those years when I was running around. Fifteen years to witness the births of my grandchildren. Fifteen years to spend time with my kids as I never did while they were growing up. Some might call that lucky, but I call that a gift. A gift from God, sure. But also a gift from those doctors. My body is my gift back to them.

As you examine me here in Gross Anatomy, I would like you to do a few things. When you look at the scars on my hands, remember I was a butcher for 45 years. When you examine my liver, remember I was a drinker. When you hold my heart in your hands, remember how I ate and my quadruple bypass. But most of all, when you are with me, learn, so that you too may be able to keep giving the gift that I was given.

I would like to thank Douglas Reifler, MD, for his support, encouragement, and insight.

Mrs Rodell

Adria Burrows, MD

People often ask me why I chose ophthalmology as my specialty. I state the reason quite simply: "Mrs Rodell."

I met Mrs Rodell when I was in medical school. I had wanted to earn some extra money; perusing the ads in the local paper, I read: "Intelligent, blind widow needs someone to read to her a few hours a week. Special interest in topics of medicine. Excellent compensation." A few hours a week seemed reasonable and wouldn't cut into my study time too seriously. I wondered why was she interested in medicine. Was she a physician? I called and scheduled an interview.

Mrs Rodell lived in a huge redbrick house in a nice section of town. A maid answered the door; she led me upstairs to a large bedroom with lace curtains and oriental rugs. Mrs Rodell sat in an immense, four-poster bed and was propped up with several plump pillows. She wore a cashmere sweater over her nightgown. As I walked in she held out a frail hand, but didn't look at me, her eyes staring blankly ahead. I took her hand and sat on the edge of the bed.

"So. You are here," Mrs Rodell said with a smile. "Tell me about yourself." I shrugged and told her I was a medical student who loved literature as well as science, so her ad had caught my eye. "Do you read or write literature?" Both. She nodded. "My husband was a physician. I always enjoyed hearing about his patients, his cures, his tragedies. Ah, and now you are the new bud entering his world . . . or what used to be his world. Maybe you'll find a cure for my disease." She turned toward me. "I have macular degeneration in both eyes. Do you want to be an ophthalmologist by any chance?" I answered no. At that time the eye didn't interest me.

I visited Mrs Rodell three times a week. I read her the newspaper and the classics and described my classes. She enjoyed hearing about my professors and my labs. She was always sitting up in her bed when I arrived, and only occasionally did she sit in a chair by her window.

Soon I began to read to her from my medical texts, and our time together became a study session. She liked psychiatry in particular and, of course, ophthalmology. There wasn't much information about macular degeneration, and I could find nothing on how to reverse progression of it.

"I hemorrhaged in the backs of my eyes," Mrs Rodell would often say. "Does the book say anything about reversing bleeding?" The answer was always no, no matter which text I had taken from the school library.

One day I made my usual trip to the house, carrying a new ophthalmology book with a long chapter on macular degeneration. The maid answered the door, but instead of pointing upstairs as she usually did, she nodded toward the end of the hall. I followed her nod, came to a thick oak door, and knocked. Mrs Rodell called, "Come in."

She was sitting in a massive, dark red, leather chair in a room lined with bookshelves. All four walls, floor to ceiling, were laden with books. Mrs Rodell was smiling proudly, as if anticipating my awe of the room. All the volumes were medical books, some very old and obviously quite valuable.

"You've never seen such a room in a house, have you? My husband was an avid collector, as was his father before him. Some of the books are from the early 19th century." As if sensing my respect for the books, she went on. "You can open any one you'd like and read to me. Our sessions will be held here from now on. You have been so good for me, you know, setting my thoughts on fire again with your reading and talk of medical school. I am alive when you come." She paused. "These books are at your disposal at any time, my dear. Use them and learn from them."

I selected a dusty tome entitled *Proposal for the Circulation of the Human Body*. What a collection!

"My husband's books cover everything . . . the eye, the ear, the gut. What subject shall we choose today? Did you notice the catalog on the right?" Her husband had arranged the titles in a file drawer by topic and author. Obviously he had taken great pride in his collection. "One thing about books," Mrs Rodell continued, "they are always waiting and willing to come to life and educate you any time you pick one up."

I was happy at that moment. Happy to see Mrs Rodell sitting away from her bedroom, happy at my new privilege to use this fine library. Imagine . . . an entire library like this at my disposal.

Even when I wasn't scheduled to read to Mrs Rodell I would bring my books to her library and supplement them with Dr Rodell's when I studied. The library became my hideaway, so to speak. I would go there almost every day and sit for hours at the enormous oak desk that dominated the room. At times I could smell the sweetness of pipe smoke. Yes, he had smoked a pipe too.

In time, Mrs Rodell had me read to her less and less often. When I did read—even if the topic was ophthalmology—her patience at sitting seemed to wane. She would cough or squirm or sigh, then announce that the session had ended. I knew she wasn't well when we returned once again to her bedroom for our sessions.

She looked pale and coughed often. Heart failure? I wondered. Pneumonia? Once I reached out to touch her forehead, thinking she had a fever, but she pushed my hand away, telling me to stop being silly. I worried about her. Finally, after I discovered she hadn't eaten in three days, I asked her maid to call an ambulance.

As Mrs Rodell sat on the gurney she reached for me. "You'll see. I'll be back tomorrow. Do use his books even when I'm not here." She squeezed me.

Mrs Rodell died of a heart attack three days later. I was not at her side. I was in her library, studying for a pathology final. The room smelled sweeter that day, of pipe tobacco. I attributed it to the warm weather.

She had had the foresight and generosity to leave me the books in her will. She worded her last testament as follows: "To my cherished reader, my educator, the one who put breath in my lungs again: I leave Dr Rodell's books and desk. May you become a great doctor and healer and never forget our times together."

I occasionally drive by the old house and look at the windows that marked her bedroom and her library. And sometimes, when I'm reading through one of her books, I can smell the sweet pipe tobacco and hear her asking, "Which topic will it be today? And why not ophthalmology?"

Tears

Paula S. Krauser, MD, MA

Brother Paul! look!
—but he rushes to a different
window.
The moon!

I heard shrieks and thought:
What's that?
That's just Suzanne
talking to the moon!
Pounding on the window
with both fists:
   Paul!   Paul!

—and talking to the moon.
Shrieking
and pounding the glass
with both fists!

Brother Paul! the moon!

William Carlos Williams, *Suzanne*

I met Danny nine years ago. This 3-year-old's face was as pale as the blond curls matted to his sweat-drenched forehead. His thin arms propped him up as he bent forward chasing his next breath. By the time I had rotated onto pediatrics, three months after Danny's admission, everyone, including Danny, had accepted his fate—he was going to die. Abnormal cells had leaked out of his kidneys and invaded his lungs, tearing apart the delicate honeycombed tissue and causing him to spew blood with every coughing spasm.

As a new intern, I was chosen to play a role in only the last scene of this tragedy. Without benefit of having known Danny before he had reached this terminal state, I felt I was an intruder, and, since I had been told there was nothing more that could be done, I felt most like an impotent imposter. I cringed whenever his mother called me "Doctor"; apparently she wanted me to feel at ease. With the help of their religion and the support of the oncology social worker, Danny's family had obviously found peace. It had been a long, painful process, but they had finally given up their beautiful son to this disease. As for me, I had not yet arrived at this point of acceptance. I was angry, frustrated, and very sad. Only Danny's mother seemed to sense that I was being forced to find my way through this maze of emotions too rapidly, and without proper preparation. Her kindness only made me feel all the more guilty and useless.

I tried to follow the lead set by my superiors, who were avoiding all unnecessary contact with Danny. But this defense only made my anguish more intense. I sought my comfort in trying to comfort Danny. At night, when the ward was quiet, I would rub his head and hold the emesis basin while he coughed. Thankfully, unlike the first few times I had tried to help, he no longer begged me to make the coughing and bleeding stop. He knew I did not have that power, knew I would cry again if he began begging.

My seasoned attending physician offered me no words of wisdom to help me cope with this difficult situation. Instead, he chastised me for doing "nurses' work" and warned me I would lose the family's respect if I did not change my behavior.

During the days that followed, I tried to act "more like a physician." I was acutely aware that my every move was being monitored and judged. I struggled to be less spontaneous, to be in control, to avoid the controversy I felt I was causing.

I failed again. As an intern, I was charged with drawing arterial blood gases. When I approached Danny with the syringe, he would retreat to the corner of his crib; it required three adults to hold him still. Since I was no longer allowed to nurture Danny, I became merely his unwilling tormentor.

I tried to imagine his wrist was attached to one of the disembodied plastic limbs on which I had practiced venipuncture. But his pulse was strong, his skin warm and soft, his whimpering a constant reminder that I was invading a living being—a little boy the same age as my own towheaded son.

To make matters worse, I became convinced this torture was unnecessary. Danny was a no code. His pale blue lips and nail beds made obtaining blood gas values superfluous. But my requests to have this procedure discontinued were met with further personal attacks. "Perhaps you should reconsider your chosen profession. Your involvement is interfering with your judgment. Maybe you don't have the stomach for this work."

Tears flowed all the more now during discussions with teachers, as my tension mounted. I wanted to rip out my lacrimal glands, those organs that were my handicap, the outward sign of my inner weakness. The attendings seemed more sympathetic to the residents who were using alcohol or other drugs to escape reality than they were to me. To them, tears were intolerable and became the focus of my evaluations, overshadowing otherwise excellent case management. To me, this crying was a reaction to the constant academic pressure, the turmoil of dealing with a dying child, the unending fatigue and the frustration of having to keep my opinions to myself—of having to fit the image, so foreign to me, of the confident, all-knowing, always-in-charge physician. Weren't tears a more appropriate outlet than screaming at nurses, being brusque with patients, or using drugs? To "them," my tears announced to the world that I was ill-equipped to be a physician, yet no one could point to one incident during which I had performed inadequately because of my "handicap." I wasted hours wondering if they were right.

Much has happened since that time, nine years ago. Part of me was stubborn enough to stick it out and believe I could be a good physician. I was lucky enough to find other interns who shared similar doubts and concerns, and together we helped each other grow. I was not unstable, as one of my attendings had suggested, but I would admit to being unable to completely suppress, or repress, my emotions. I still cry too easily. I still get frustrated and angry when I feel helpless, still irritable when I am exhausted and overworked. I still feel very vulnerable. All that has changed is the context.

Currently, as a physician in private practice, I find I have been able to deal with the realities of life and illness better than I dealt with the daily process of medical education. My patients judge me less harshly than my professors used to. Rather than assuming my tears are signs of weakness, my patients tend to see them as my way of acknowledging that we share the vicissitudes of the human condition and that they are not alone in their sorrow.

I rarely have to pound the window with both fists now.

The Intern's Vein

Jordan Smoller, MD

I was just finishing a note when the senior resident pulled me aside. "There's a lady in room 9 with a probable DVT. Go ahead and get an IV in her, get her bloods off, and start getting a history. I'll be there in a few minutes."

It was the spring of my fourth year in medical school, and the threat of internship was looming large. This emergency room rotation was to be my last clinical rotation before graduation, and I was determined to master some of the minor procedures that I needed to feel comfortable with before my student days were over. Like putting in IVs. In a couple of months I'd be a doctor, and it would be just too embarrassing to ask for help with something as simple as that.

I gathered up my IV kit, strode into the examining room, and introduced myself as one of the medical students. Mrs Tannenbaum was an obese white female in no apparent distress. "Hello, Doctor," she said, looking up at me anxiously.

"Can you tell me what's brought you in to the emergency room?"

"Dr Sanderson told me to come here."

"And why was that?" I asked absently, scanning her hands for a suitable vein.

"Well, I went to clinic because last Thursday I felt this lump under my arm and my leg started swelling up and—"

"Keep talking. I'm just going to put in an IV and draw a little blood," I said as I tied a tourniquet around her left wrist. Her eyes widened and she stared at her hand with a worried look. "Go on, you were saying that your leg was hurting . . ."

"No, my uh, my leg was swelling and Dr Sanderson looked at it and said I should come to the emergency room. Am I going to have to stay in the hospital?"

"Well, we don't know for sure yet. When did the leg start to . . . uh (*There's a good one on the back of her hand.*) . . . start to swell?" I asked as I put the angiocath in. She pulled away slightly. I wasn't getting any blood return. I retreated and tried to advance the catheter again. Nothing.

"I don't know, I guess on Sunday." Her eyes were fixed on her hand as I kept poking. She continued with her story: she had lost 15 pounds over the past month and had found a lump in her right axilla. Three days later her left calf had become swollen and red. (*There we go—a flash of blood in the IV. Now advance the catheter. Damn. I lost it.*) "You remind me of my son."

"Oh really? What does your son do?" I asked in a friendly tone, hoping I could distract her from my fumbling with a little small talk.

"He's an engineer. He lives in California with his wife."

"Uh-huh." (*Forget it. This one's blown.*) "Do you see much of him?"

"No. He hasn't come to Boston in seven years. He works very hard. They're real busy. . . . Did you get it yet?"

"No. I'm afraid we're going to have to try again on the other side," I said matter-of-factly, as though this kind of thing happens all the time.

"That's okay, Doctor," she said gently. "I just hope I don't have to stay. I don't like this hospital."

"Why's that?" I asked, slapping her right hand to try to get a rise out of her veins.

"The last time I was here was 17 years ago . . . with my husband."

"Mmmmm." I could see only one thready-looking vein, but I decided to go for it.

"Ow!" she started, but then caught herself. I could feel her looking at my eyes, but I was focused on her hand. "We were married 24 years. He was coughing and coughing for months. And one day, he coughed up blood and I took him down here to the emergency room. He didn't want to go." (*Wait a minute. There's a flash . . . and . . .*)

"When the doctor came out—I was in that waiting room out there. I knew it was bad news. He told me to sit down." (*I think I'm in!*) "He said . . . 'It's cancer' and . . ." She stopped. (*Oh great, resistance. Pull back.*) "Are you getting it?"

"Not yet. Sorry this is taking so long," I said warmly. I heard my own voice and its "warmth" suddenly sounded so professional. I advanced again. (*I don't believe this! Another one blown.*) Without even trying to explain myself, I pulled out, retied the tourniquet around her forearm, and opened a third angiocath. Time to go for the intern's vein.

I glanced at Mrs Tannenbaum. She looked lost, frightened. "I've got to get home tonight," she said, and I thought I heard her voice tremble.

"Is there somebody waiting for you at home?" I asked as I stroked her wrist with an alcohol swab.

"Oh, no." She paused. "I've been alone since Gabe died."

"Oh. I'm sorry."

"He was the only man I've ever been with. There's no one who could take his place. He was my angel. He . . . I loved him so much." Her voice choked.

I looked up and saw her face—really for the first time. I saw her thin curls of hair, still a few strands of blond among the gray. Her soft face was moist with perspiration. Her sad eyes caught mine, and they suddenly seemed so familiar. I imagined an old photograph, black-and-white and worn. A younger Mrs Tannenbaum in a flowing ivory gown with a handsome young man in a dinner jacket. Those eyes so filled with love as she looked up at him. I thought of my own fiancée and remembered how she had awakened me this morning with a gentle kiss.

"I was at this hospital every day. They wouldn't let me sleep in his room, but I brought him his favorite soup and fed him every day. Near the end he couldn't eat." I thought of my father as he lay in a hospital bed, a week from his death. His face was gaunt and pale, his legs edematous. My mother petting his forehead. He looked up at her and overcame his near-delirium long enough to say, "I love you." My mother's eyes filled with tears and his glazed over again as the morphine and hypercalcemia overtook him.

"He always took care of me," Mrs Tannenbaum continued. "I was here on his last night. He was so weak, he could barely move. He took my hand and put it up to his mouth, and . . . I thought he was going to kiss me. He put his lips on my wedding ring and . . ." She stopped and looked away, her lips quivering. "He slid the ring off with his lips and he . . . he swallowed it."

There in room 9, with tears in our eyes, I held Mrs Tannenbaum's hand. And we both thought of her husband and the unfathomable beauty of his farewell to her. In that one gesture he had taken the symbol of their love inside him so it would forever be a part of him—but in that same moment, he had freed her. Because he loved her so deeply, he was telling her to go on with her life and to find love again. Mrs Tannenbaum and I looked at each other for a long time without saying a word.

Finally, I looked down again at the angiocath in my other hand, and as I held her hand, I slipped the IV into the intern's vein. A flash of blood. I was in. The senior resident stuck his head into the room. "Did you get it?" he asked.

I looked at Mrs Tannenbaum. "Yes," I answered softly.

When to Touch

Diane Morse, MD

I had been called about the patient before. She was a young woman, in her 20s, with AIDS. She'd been hospitalized most recently because of intractable seizures, probably secondary to toxoplasmosis and lymphoma. The last time I was on call, her seizures were being treated with diazepam, and I was asked to cross-cover at night for her regular resident physician because she was still seizing. I went to her room and encountered her mother, who was clearly distraught. She begged me to tell her whether the end was near, whether she should stay the night. I didn't know what to say; although I sensed her daughter's death wasn't imminent, I couldn't promise. I told her this. She seemed incredibly despondent, but I had other calls to answer and asked the nurse to try to console her.

A few days later, I was again called about the patient. She was a "no code," and she had died. Would I, as resident physician on call, come and "pronounce" her?

Throughout my nine months of internship, this practice has seemed strange to me, each time I am called to do it. The nurses, the family, everyone in the room can plainly see that someone is dead. Am I there to give official sanction, to comfort, to discuss organ donation, to request an autopsy permit, to perform a ritual? It has never really been clear to me. Each time I walk in and check the pulse, pupils, respirations, heart— all eyes on me, some already tearful. Frequently there is relief mixed with sadness, when a long-suffering loved one finally dies.

That night, I went into the room and saw the mother stretched out across her daughter, holding her and weeping aloud. This was the first time I had seen someone hold or even touch the newly dead person. At first, I felt like an intruder. This was the outraged grief of a mother losing her young, healthy, beautiful daughter to a terrible disease. Could I be unobtrusive? Impossible, with the mother practically lying on the bed, covering her child. Could I comfort her? Her grief seemed endless—and private. Yet I often have the feeling, as a physician, that I'm walking into private areas. A friend from medical school once chided me for failing to ask necessary questions that I thought were too nosy.

I walked in and touched the mother on the shoulder. She stood and faced me, tears streaming down her face. She said, "Oh, Doctor, I remember you. It's happened so fast. . . ." Clumsily I tried to touch her, to comfort her, and then suddenly I was holding the crying mother close. She began to tell me stories about her daughter; my beeper remained blessedly silent. She told me about when her daughter first became blind with CMV retinitis and nervously asked the time at frequent intervals. Soon the mother began to tell her the time without being asked, until finally her daughter got a braille watch. It became a private joke, she told me, for the daughter to tell her the time many times a day. It was her way of saying, "Thank you for reassuring me when I was scared. I'm OK now." As she told the stories she kept touching her daughter: her hands, her face, her arms. She continued to cry, not seeming to mind that I too wiped my eyes a few times.

What was different for me about this death? Was it the patient's age? Her diagnosis? Her mother's open sadness and mourning? Perhaps, but I think what made it touch me was allowing myself to feel for the surviving relative, something I don't usually do. If I had died, my mother would cry like this one. Seeing my mother in her, I felt a new sadness and caring. I'm still experimenting with what's "right" to do as a doctor, and I feel it was "right" to involve myself this time. This mother needed someone to share her grief and horror about her child and the never-imagined disease from which she had just died. As a developing physician I'm learning that privacy can be respected too much, and that sometimes closeness is needed, even when it hurts.

Healing Arts

Lisa M. Lanzarone, MD

The ritual that gets me through the day starts with a jolt from REM sleep. First sound of the day: static from the clock-radio. First thought: another day of this dehumanizing internship. First sight: a whitewashed, empty face in the mirror. This is me.

My mind has abandoned its search for meaning in my work on the medical wards. The Fraternity that is Medicine, like all the others, requires that members must survive rituals of pain before they can enter the fold. But the human organism knows that repeated trauma causes the skin to lose sensation; the only protection is respite, which is not my privilege this morning. I cannot recall exactly when I gave up the search and wonder if numbness has begun to shape my thoughts.

Still, internship is only a year, almost half over; residency will be an improvement. By then I might enjoy leading everyone on work rounds: an endless exercise in which mobs of house staff and medical students converge at 6 AM on the sleepy and infirm. "How was your night, sir?" "Have you passed any gas yet?" From such data, key medication changes will be made. Our medical successes often seem excesses: witness the diabetic smoker who survived several heart attacks in order to experience the piecemeal amputation of limbs starved by the original disease. Or cut to the steelworker with emphysema, found unconscious by neighbors and whose sole misfortune was his neglect to carry a living will in his back pocket. He remains unaware of his surroundings, his voice kept silent by the endotracheal tube that has become an appendage, weeks after his arrival. The art of healing lies buried under a morass of cure.

Five-fifteen. Just enough time to splash water onto my sleep-encrusted eyes and shuffle through a lifeless wardrobe. My ritual of self-healing begins again this morning with 20 slices of Wonder Bread, two rows across, each slopped with a spoonful of peanut butter and jelly. Out the door at 5:45 with no time to waste. In the harsh cold, I think of a woman, an old black homeless unknown with arachnoid fingers and a face wrinkled against the wind like an ancient tribal chief's. Her image stays before me as I move along, by the five or so unkempt panhandlers strewn among their niches along the few blocks to the hospital.

The PBJs reach their destinations quietly, as I tuck them into the sour wraps of these sleepy vagrants, who will remain unconscious until the first sunlight stings their swollen eyelids. Manageable by even the shakiest hands, with a simplicity of design only a mother could invent, the sandwiches qualify as the perfect food. These pasty creations are high-octane fuel: sugar for the heavy drinkers who will wake up hung over and hypoglycemic; protein, sorely needed by all; and vitamins (Wonder Bread is the only brand that tastes like a multivitamin), partly thiamine and folate, for the delirious who mingle about, talking trash to curbside Buicks, in neurologic fits from deficiencies. One can only guess how people end up as litter on the sidewalk. In the dark and cold I succumb to familiar sensations of fatigue and inadequacy, if only for a moment, as I wonder how these elders became my charges. Was it something my parents taught me as a child, or is this some form of compensation for the impotence that stifles the motions of my hours and days as an intern in this system?

On this sidewalk, however, I command the service; as usual, I have extra sandwiches for the woman with the spidery hands, who is usually the last one I encounter. Asleep she is rather lovely, her thin arms shielding threadbare dreams from cold night air. I sense that she has nurtured many, and will need the extra energy to sustain herself. In sleep she is unaware that in receiving my offering, she nurtures yet another. If I had the nerve to wake her, I would tell her this, and much, much more.

Bending to tuck the sandwiches into her arms, I see no steam near her face, unlike the others in fitful sleep. And I can't satisfy myself that her chest rises and falls with life, as she is embalmed in layers of worn woolens. My heart begins to race, as she is pulseless, at both the wrist and the neck. She is stiff and cold to the touch, but January spares none of us. Finally, I shake her; she does not awaken.

Stepping back, I see she looks more rested than the others. Her eyes are closed; she must have died in her sleep. The permanence of her night's sleep is almost enviable. I resist the reflex to breathe into her mouth. Was it for her sake or for mine that I thought of trying to resuscitate her lifeless body? And if she survived such efforts, would she ever be able to speak for herself? Looking at her here, it seems not.

But the questions linger, along with the handful of sticky sandwiches that will be my dinner, nourishing an image that refuses to fade in the brightly lit mecca of medicine ahead. Ambling toward the phone booth to notify the police of the body, I am simultaneously warmed and made numb by my decision, which motioned to me from a distant corner of logic. All this time that logic had been obscured by the harsh tint of those hospital lights. Finally, on a cold, dark sidewalk, I can feel the shape of its boundaries.

Ten past six. I will be late for morning rounds.

The Legacy

John C. Cozart, MD

My last doctor was a real jerk, and I bet you will be too!"

That concluded my first conversation with Phil. I was starting my second month of internship, my first day on the cancer service. I had walked from room to room, introducing myself to all of the patients, and had found Phil sound asleep. A sign posted over his bed read: "CAUTION—DAY SLEEPER!" I shook Phil awake and quickly realized I had made a mistake.

"Can't you read, you idiot?" he yelled. "That sign's up there for a reason!" He went on to inform me that his opinion of doctors, *especially* interns, was very low. "I sleep until at least noon each day, and don't you forget it!"

Phil was six feet two and muscular, with piercing blue eyes. He was 19 and back in the hospital with another relapse of acute lymphocytic leukemia. As a result of chemotherapy, he sported only a few wisps of blond hair. As the days passed, I found myself spending as much time with him as I could. I answered his questions and explained the results of his numerous tests.

One day I asked Phil what his life had been like before he became sick. "Before this leukemia got me down, I used to ride a Harley and party all night," he told me. "I could drink a six-pack of beer in less than three minutes."

Phil really came alive at night. Dressed in his favorite Guns N' Roses T-shirt and armed with a high-powered water gun shaped like an M-16, Phil terrorized the nurses. One night, while I was examining another patient, I heard screams in the hall. Looking out the door, I saw one of the nurses, her face already drenched with water, receive one last blast before Phil slipped back into his room.

Phil's mother worked at a local factory and spent all of her free time at his side. She slept on a cot in the corner of his room.

"Mom," I overheard Phil complain another night, "I just can't stop throwing up from the chemotherapy. Even the special medicines for nausea don't help."

"I know, baby. Just close your eyes and try to relax," she whispered in his ear. "This cool cloth on your forehead will help you go to sleep." Small and frail, she held his huge body in her arms, and the retching finally passed.

Two weeks later a striking brunet came to visit Phil. Tall and slender with green eyes, she spent most of the afternoon with him. I wondered who she was.

Phil, exhausted from the visit, was sound asleep. I noticed the sign above his bed had been amended: "INTERNS WILL BE SHOT ON SIGHT!" I gently nudged Phil awake and asked, "Who was the green-eyed beauty?"

"Now, Doc, you may not be as big a jerk as I first thought, but there's some information I just can't give out. It's for me to know and you to dream about."

"I see you added another warning," I nodded toward his sign.

"And it means what it says!" Without warning Phil whipped out the water gun from under his bed. A blast of cold water caught me on the cheek as I fled the room and his raucous laughter.

Later that night I asked his mother who the girl was.

"That's Lucy, his girlfriend. I think his happiest moments are during his visits from her."

Early one morning a week later, I was rounding with my attending in Phil's room. "So, how are you this morning?" the attending asked.

"I knew that intern couldn't read. I guess you're illiterate as well!"

"What did you say?" the attending demanded. In response, Phil flipped a switch on his enormous boom box: "Highway to Hell" by AC/DC screeched at full volume. As Phil started to sing along, the attending's face turned beet red with anger, and I struggled to stifle my laughter. Later that day, I went back to see Phil.

"I'm sorry that I was such a jerk this morning," he said. "It's just that living in this hospital is such a drag. My friends have quit coming to see me."

"What about your girlfriend?" I asked.

He paused, then said quietly, "She said it's too hard to be around somebody who's dying." He looked away and ran a hand over his head. "I don't even have any hair."

At that moment I finally understood who Phil really was. Beneath that outrageous, exasperating exterior was just a scared boy, alone, afraid of dying. Gently, I placed my arm around his shoulders, hoping he wouldn't shrug it off.

"I wish there was a cure for leukemia," he whispered.

"I do too, Phil. I do too."

After that, Phil often invited me to his room to listen to tapes. "I've always wanted to play guitar," he confessed one day, "and I'd just started to play with a band when I got sick."

He liked to play his radio loud, close his eyes, and strum along on his guitar. I think he must have imagined himself on-stage, before a huge audience, in a world far away from sickness and disease. I wanted to give him that world, to make sure that he never came back to mine.

Phil was finally discharged during my last week on the cancer service. As I walked into his room to say good-bye, I spotted him picking up the water gun. Quickly I ducked for cover.

"Hey, don't worry," he said. "I won't shoot you. I'm going home today and won't have much use for this thing. It worked real well on you—got you in shape. Why don't I just leave it with you, so you can blast the nurses if they get out of line?" I promised him I would take good care of it.

Three nights later, after an especially busy night on call, I was finally able to lie down. My beeper went off 15 minutes later.

"John, I just got a call from a local hospital." It was the oncology fellow. "Phil's at their emergency room with a fever and low WBC count. They're transferring him here. He should be here in about an hour."

I wiped the sleep from my eyes, grabbed some coffee, and tried to remember the workup for neutropenic fever. Forty-five minutes later, one of the nurses, frantic, ran up to me.

"Our emergency room just called. Phil went into asystole in the ambulance about 15 minutes ago. He's in the ER being coded."

"Does Phil's mother know?"

"No. She's still on her way here."

I found Phil lying on the table, intubated, his young body jerking with each chest compression. For a moment he seemed to breathe on his own, then there was nothing. I glanced at the ECG monitor and saw only a flat line. We tried everything to revive him, but it was useless.

I left the ER, exhausted, and suddenly realizing that Phil's mother was still on her way to the hospital. How could I tell her that her son had died?

A few minutes later she walked up to me at the nurses' station. I knew immediately that she understood what had happened by the stricken look on my face.

"I'm so sorry. Phil's gone," I said. "I just wish I could have done more for him."

"Doctor, I know you loved my baby, and he knew it too. And that's as good as any medicine you could have given him."

As I watched Phil's mother slowly walk away, I felt a tap on my shoulder. It was the head nurse.

"I'm sorry to bother you, but it's Billy," she announced. "He's here for induction chemotherapy. All the nurses have tried but we can't stop him from crying."

Grabbing a plastic bag from behind the nurses' station, I followed her into a room. Lying face down on his bed was an 8-year-old child, softly sobbing.

"Hi, Billy. My name's John," I offered.

"I *hate* it here!" he cried, burying his face deeper into the pillow. "There's nothing to play with. And that lady in the white dress? She just stuck a big needle in me! Why can't you just leave me alone?"

"Billy," I pressed, "I had a very special friend who gave me a present before he left the hospital."

"Who *cares*?" He was quiet for a moment, then curiosity got the best of him. He peeped up at me, then his eyes widened as I held out Phil's giant water gun.

"My friend Phil used to shoot the nurses when they got out of line. Sometimes he would even shoot me. This helped him get through some tough times, and I think he would have wanted you to have it. Would you like to give it a try?"

Shreds of a Flowered Shirt

Emily R. Transue

I watched someone die today.

It's the first week of Medicine, my first rotation. We're in the middle of morning rounds when a code blue blasts suddenly over the pager. The patient is coming in by ambulance in ten minutes, time enough for a carefully unhurried walk to the ED.

The team stands in readiness in the resuscitation room. I linger by the ambulance entrance, watching the still-quiet drive, the softly falling rain.

Finally the ambulance pulls up, lights whirling. The stretcher emerges with the patient (we know it's a woman, about 60 years old), feet first, legs slightly apart, thin, deathly white, and naked.

The EMTs wheel her in. A swarm of medical personnel descends instantly: intubating, inserting IVs, sticking on leads, attaching monitors, calling for shock: "Charging, everybody clear? One, two, three—" The body lurches on the table; all eyes fix on the ECG screen.

"Some epi . . . " A flutter (if you can have a flutter, superimposed on chaos), needles, vials, tubes. A vial drops on the floor, the sound of breaking glass. Someone kicks it under the cart.

Words fly across the table responding to blips on the screen: V-tach, V-fib, asystole; others I don't catch. Periodically CPR is halted for a few seconds and everyone reaches to feel for a pulse, hope outweighing the evidence of the ECG. "I have something . . ." someone cries occasionally; then a moment later, "Gone . . ." "Agonal rhythm," Steve, my resident, says matter-of-factly.

Shreds of a flowered shirt dangle from the table (I'd heard they cut your clothes off when you had a cardiac arrest, but never really knew): pitiful remnants of personhood.

She is naked. After a while someone drapes a towel over her exposed genitals, but it quickly falls off again and no one bothers to replace it. I am too frightened to—frightened of what? Of the body, of being seen as "soft"?

Steve (we, the students, love Steve, we want to become Steve) officiates, under the watchful eye of the ED attending. He is calm and competent, a walking manual of proper code blue protocol.

At first they don't even know who she is: "No ID," reports the ambulance team. "No ID? Anything? A purse?" The word "purse," emanating from the lips of these sterile scrubs-clad ED personnel in this bleak white room full of sharp metallic instruments, is oddly out of place, a lay object evinced in this utterly medicalized world. What kind of a purse did she have, this woman, back when she was a woman, before she became only a body? A tight black leather clutch with a folding flap and gold metal buckle? A bright basket-weave bag?

But later—oddly soon, in fact, after the cry of "No ID"—they have not only a name but a chart: this body has CAD, CHF, a history of lymphoma. Her daughters are here—Ah, at last, a confirmation of those shreds of flowered cloth, this WAS a person after all. Daughters. Somewhere in a hallway are daughters waiting to hear that their mother is dead, maybe not knowing yet what all but the greenest of us (meaning me—but even I knew) have known from the beginning, that this exercise in resuscitation is a futile one. Daughters who will weep and grieve and someday heal.

Someone, mercifully, closes the door.

When the CPR team is tired, Steve says, "Med students, you want to do compressions?" I nod, put on gloves (one tears, as I pull it on), step in. From above I can see for the first time her face, albeit deformed by the tape holding the intubation tube in place, her curly graying hair. Her eyes are open. What is she feeling? I wonder. Anything? I find myself hoping fervently that her brain is dead already from lack of oxygen. Dear God, when I die, don't let them do all this to me— Meanwhile I am thrusting on her chest, firm and fast, over and over. "Faster," someone says, and I speed the pulses. Her rib cage is resilient, neither rigid nor relaxed, but moves satisfyingly under my pressure. I am irrationally concerned with not breaking her ribs. "Good compressions," they say approvingly. "You can feel the pulse." They will repeat this later, as if to console me, as if it made any difference; what matter good compressions or no, she was dead anyway.

The new intern does compressions until he is clearly exhausted, but he will not complain—later I will be the same way, refusing relief even when a nurse suggests it, holding out to the bitter end: "I'm calling it," says Steve. "Anyone object to my calling it?" Silence. Everyone steps away from the body. There is no moment of last respect, only a rush for the sink as gloves are tossed into the wastebasket. The body is forgotten. It lies on the stretcher, only an obstacle now to be pushed aside on the way to the sink, the new center of attention, cleanliness, departure, sanity.

Others come to cover the corpse—officially a corpse, at last, no longer that strange, pale, intermediate object, neither alive nor dead—with a cloth.

Somewhere daughters are being told that their mother is dead, the final shreds of hope being torn away. A harrowing day for them, the daughters; the dread call from the hospital ("We're sorry, something has happened—"), the breathless over-the-speed-limit drive, double-parking in the ED lot. Waiting helplessly, clinging together, in sterile foreign hallways, trying to be strong, "for her." "We're doing our best," they're told. "But we have to be honest with you, it doesn't look good." And now the doctor comes to confirm their worst fears. I don't know who tells them; so many doctors rushing in and out, no one leaps out at me as being the One. I would like to ask, even to go with him, to meet the daughters; to grasp with something more than torn flowered cloth the humanity of this body, this person who is the first I have seen die. But my team is going, and I need them, Steve, my intern, the other medical student, some semblance of security. And I don't realize until too late that what I want is to go and offer my sorrow to the daughters, in so doing to get back perhaps a little of my own humanity.

And the code has made me late. I have to run to get to conference by noon.

Portraits

John D. Rowlett, MD

Early one Sunday morning, even before I had the chance to change into my scrubs, I received a stat page to the emergency room. I was only a few months into my internship, and though I was becoming familiar with routine calls, stat pages had a tendency to mean runs of V-tach— mine. I arrived at the emergency room simultaneously with the ambulance. A 2-year-old, found unresponsive by her parents, lay motionless on the gurney. She had been intubated by the paramedics, but her heart had failed to respond. Despite prolonged CPR, countless rounds of drugs, endless fluids, and a temporary pacemaker, the young heart remained silent. Reluctantly, I stopped the code.

Explaining these events to Christy's parents was one of the most difficult experiences of my young career. Fortunately, the attending, who had supervised both the attempted resuscitation and my conversation, recognized my struggle. "You handled everything well," he reassured me. "You know, I've been to hundreds of arrests in this emergency room. You get better at dealing with them, but a child's death is always painful." Sensing my distress, he continued. "Sometimes I jog as a way to escape the hospital—maybe it would work for you."

I was too tired to run, but a friend had given me a camera as a graduation gift—now seemed a good time to learn how to use it. The spectacular scenery of nearby Lake Michigan allows even inexperienced photographers like me to take a fairly good picture. The next evening, while thinking of Christy, I took a picture of an old lighthouse. The photo turned out a bit hazy, but to this day it hangs on a wall in my bedroom.

During the next three years there were many more calls to the emergency room, more codes, and more pictures. With time, my pictures, each a vivid reminder of a shortened life, improved. Likewise, my ability to handle a crisis grew. Yet, like my teacher, I struggled with each death, with each new picture on the wall.

On a snowy day in my third year I was again called to the ER. The helicopter was to land in just a few minutes and the PICU team had been requested. As we made our way to the pad, the dispatcher gave me the scant available information. "Lethargic 2-year-old boy with fever and rash. Blood pressure is better after fluid bolus but perfusion is still poor. One peripheral IV. We're the nearest PICU with any bed space. Three minutes to arrival."

As the chopper landed, the team rushed to the small child. He was minimally arousable, hypotensive, and tachycardic. His airway was patent but he was tiring.

Once in the ICU he was intubated and received the necessary lines. Bags of IV fluids, antibiotics, and inotropes took their place beside the ventilator. As the labs returned and the numbers deteriorated, it became clear his chances were bleak. I hoped we could support him at least until his family traveled the 90 miles between hospitals.

Two hours later his weary parents arrived. Both college students, they listened as I tried to explain the situation. Together they struggled to understand why their son, so healthy only a day before, was likely to die of a disease called meningococcemia. In the back of my mind I knew that tomorrow I would need to buy film before heading to the lake.

Miraculously, the child survived the night. Still, the next evening I drove to the beach. There, memories of previous such trips and the simple pictures that now covered a wall dominated my thoughts. The lake was frozen; the sky, dreary. Yet, in winter's tomb, I found the escape I so needed.

The next morning I returned to the ICU. Anthony was still alive, but his problems were increasing. The penicillin had begun to kill the meningococcus, but the resulting disseminated intravascular coagulation waged war on his young body. He hemorrhaged into his lungs, intestinal tract, and soft tissues.

Over the next few days Anthony made small improvements. His mother never left his side—cheering each minuscule advance, ignoring the major setbacks. He began to recover from the renal failure, but I never was sure if it was the furosemide or his mother's coaching that was responsible for the diuresis. It didn't really matter. With time, the other organs began to recover from the devastation of the infection and resultant DIC. He was weaned from the ventilator and was able to tolerate small sips of orange juice. Multiple surgeries were attempted to restore his legs, ravaged by compartment syndrome. Cautiously, we began to talk about survival.

Unbelievably, the devastation of infection seemed to have spared Anthony's mind. He quickly became the center of attention as he asked for his favorite things. He seemed particularly fascinated by the snow falling outside his window.

It was snowing the morning Anthony's mother strapped him into his car seat for the long ride home. His legs were casted—an attempt to limit the contraction of his unopposed posterior muscles. Pillows and coats made a soft resting place. After a two-month stay in the hospital, he and his parents were eager to go home. Before the car pulled away I slipped an envelope to his parents. In it was a picture—the one I'd taken for their son that dreary evening months earlier. I told them I would explain later, and that I wanted Anthony to have it.

A few weeks later I received a letter from Anthony's mother. She wrote optimistically of his progress and future surgeries. She thanked me for the picture, which she had hung in Anthony's room. With her letter she enclosed a simple drawing. At first it appeared to be just another 2-year-old's scribbles that belonged on the refrigerator. But this one was special. In it I saw not simple lines but the rebirth of a human life.

This priceless drawing now hangs beside a frozen sunset on a new wall in my room—a wall dedicated to the celebration of life.

Paths

Ellen Kroop-Martin, MD

There were no clues that this was to be a memorable rotation. It was early in the academic year and my first ward rotation in the dim green halls of a southern VA hospital. I felt equal but competing surges of anxiety and anticipation. Armed for combat with a brand new "Washington manual" and blazing bright lab coat, I listened attentively as my senior resident introduced me to "our service." It seemed manageable. That is, until Mr W.

Even before I laid eyes on him, I knew Mr W was trouble. With the selfish insecurity of a new intern, I listened to his problem list. One by one the problems leapt from my resident's mouth onto my shoulders, dragging down my spirit and any hope I had for leaving the hospital that century.

Mr W had been in the hospital a long time. He had been worked up for a variety of illnesses and was on a complex array of medicines. His diagnosis was still uncertain. It was simply too much. Even as I desperately tried to listen, my mind screamed in protest: "How can I manage a man who has defied other, more experienced and capable physicians?" In my imagination, Mr W was a giant who had slain my hopes of having a successful rotation.

Already defeated, I followed my resident into the room. My "giant" was a cachectic, crotchety man. He had been through a parade of new doctors many times before and was frankly unimpressed by his newest charge. With scathing indifference, he ignored us as we did our quick bedside examination. My pounding head quieted just enough to hear my own first impression. Bending over the lowered bed rail, trying to auscultate his heart, I couldn't make a seal with the diaphragm of my stethoscope. His body was simply too wasted. The reality of that gap between my stethoscope and his skin suddenly struck me. Medical knowledge would have to wait. My first task from that minute on was to fill that ravine that divided us. This was not an eloquent or especially compassionate thought. I literally wanted to get some calories into and muscle onto this man. The thought became my life preserver on a sea of his confounding history. I needed a manageable goal and, since understanding his medical history seemed out of my range for the foreseeable future, this seemed like a good starting place.

It wasn't simple. Mr W had been in the system longer than I. Apparently, enthusiasm and good intentions were not new to him. He had weathered the storm of other interns and when they left he was still there. This seemed his only certainty. However, perhaps because I had no lofty aspirations and approached my goal tenaciously as my means of surviving, I began to wear him down.

He had not been out of his bed for most of three medical charts worth of information, nor had he been outside the hospital. So I got him a trapeze. I got him a physical therapist. I got him a wheelchair. I got to him. He used the trapeze and small miracles happened. The nurses became interested. Mr W assisted in his ADLs. And while I was still trying to sort through his medical problems and diagnostic dilemmas, this proud and aloof man gathered back some independence.

My story could probably end here, but it doesn't. My real lesson occurred the first time I wheeled Mr W outside.

I was feeling very proud of myself. Mr W was moving almost independently from bed to wheelchair, and he had gained some weight and had even been caught smiling in some nurses' reports. Smugly, I wheeled my prized patient outside. I asked him where he wanted to go. It was a beautiful fall day. In my mind, the trees were competing for the chance to shade this awesome man.

Trees didn't win that day. Mr W wanted to "sit with the boys." Sit with the boys and smoke. Smoke. Stunned, I delivered him to his requested destination and gave him his privacy.

I was crestfallen, indignant, and hurt. All of my hard work literally seemed to go up in flames. After all I had done for him, Mr W had betrayed me. I had confusedly mistaken his progress for a promise to comply with my entire health agenda. Petulant and confused, I was left to ponder his betrayal.

Several days later the lesson came to me. As physicians, all we can really do is celebrate the human spirit. Entrusted with its secrets, we delve into its mysteries, seek understanding. We tirelessly work to revive it to whatever level of function it can perform. But when all is done, it is not ours. We revive the body and hopefully the spirit, simply that it may follow its desired course. We can encourage potential paths, but the reward is not the path the patient takes, but that they were well enough to choose one.

The Chief Complaint

Ann E. Dominguez

We always hope that the last patient before lunch has a simple problem. Usually, however, the last patient before lunch is the one who needs several hours of our time and four lengthy, expensive studies before we know what to do for him. Mr L was my last patient before lunch.

I asked him, as I always ask my patients, what brought him to the clinic that day, and he couldn't remember. So I asked him what was bothering him, and he said, "Injustice." Injustice did not seem to be a problem easily managed before lunch.

I asked my question in another way. "Do you have any pain?"

"My head hurts," he replied, "because when I was 13, living in the South, a white man hit me over the head with a beer bottle." He told me the story of this attack: brutal, unprovoked, answered with a beating. I did not know what to do for 60-year-old headaches.

I nodded and asked, "Anything else?" I was a little afraid of the answer.

"I have a scar on my leg," he said, "because when I was in the army, a white doctor cut me for no reason and . . ." He recounted another story of my race's attacks on him and his people. Following this came an account of being run off the road by the white children's school bus as he walked to the black school six miles away from his home.

I have been taught to control the medical interview, but this interview was thoroughly out of my control. We had been in the examination room for a full 20 minutes, and I had no idea why he had come to the doctor or what I should do for him. I noticed my heart pounding and the feel of sweat on my forehead. "But what is bothering you *today*?" I asked, as if italics could make things clear and impress on him my desire to know his current problem.

"Injustice," he said simply.

I looked in frustration at my triage sheet. A note from the nurse jumped out at me: *Patient and helper are extremely poor historians* (code for "could not tell the nurse a good story of his illness"). On the contrary, I thought, this man is an excellent historian and had told me several stories of why he was unwell . . . but none of it was anything I could change. Time was ticking, my stomach was grumbling, and I did not know what to do.

"Somebody up there loves me," he ventured, "or I never would have made it this far."

"Oh?" I said. "Who is that?"

"Jesus," he replied. "Jesus loves me."

"He loves me too," I said. "Would you like to pray?"

Mr L leaned forward and cocked his ear toward me. "What did you say, honey? My hearing must be going after all this time."

"Would you like to pray?" I asked again. "To Jesus."

Mr L gave me a wide smile. "What kind of doctor are you? I'd love to pray!"

We bowed our heads, and Mr L began praying. I listened to his prayers about his fears and anger, about his frustration with racism and hatred, and about his aches and pains. When he had finished, I prayed for his headache, for the cold he felt in his bones, for the painful scars on his body, and for Jesus to forgive us (my people, the people in the South whom I had never met, but for whom I stood when Mr L came into my office) for hurting him and hating him. I prayed for God to end the injustice. "Amen."

"Amen," he echoed. "Thank you so much."

"Thank you," I said. My heart rate had returned to normal, and I felt I had actually done something to help this man, whose complaints I could not mend. We discussed his medications and his regular doctor, and when Mr L would visit him next. He put on his hat and started to get up from his chair, and I remembered that my preceptor needed to see him before he left. "Could you wait just a few minutes, Mr L, so my supervisor could say hello to you?"

He smiled and told me to take my time. I dashed out of the room and looked again at my triage and billing sheets. What was I going to say to my preceptor? "Chief complaint of injustice; differential diagnosis: racism, hatred, fear. Plan: prayer. Follow-up in three weeks." Hardly. There was nothing I had done for this man that Medicare would pay for.

My preceptor was in the other room waiting for me. "Ready?" she asked.

"I've had sort of a hard time with this patient," I said, as she stood and followed me back to the examination room. "He didn't really come with a physical complaint . . ."

She started from ground zero, and I watched her frustration develop, as mine had, with his nonmedical complaints. She examined him, which I had not done, and then we called his primary physician and accessed the computer for a summary of any past visits or hospital stays. His physician told us that Mr L was dying of his cancer and simply needed periodic checks that he was still functioning well at home. We returned to the room, and she asked him about his cancer, which he denied.

Eventually, she shrugged her shoulders and nodded to me. "All right, Mr L," she said, "you'll see your regular doctor in three weeks. Is everything all right at home?"

Mr L nodded and smiled. "Yes, ma'am. Thank you." Then he stood and reached for my hand. "And thank *you*," he said. "You're quite a little doctor."

We watched him walk down the hall with his cane. When he disappeared around the corner, my preceptor said, "Better get to lunch. What's your diagnosis?"

I shook my head. "Headache? Cold?"

"Write medication check, prostate cancer, dementia." She waited for me to circle the codes on the billing sheet. "Did you just talk to him? He seemed pretty happy with your visit."

My mouth went dry. "We talked about injustice," I replied. I didn't mention our prayer.

"He's a hard patient," she said. "Good job." She walked away to lunch, and I carried my billing sheets to the desk on my way to lunch.

I thought that he wasn't such a hard patient. Rather, it's a hard life, full of injustice. And he was quite a historian.

Are You Sure?

Thomas M. Gill, MD

Before she was reassigned to me, 82-year-old Mrs Hines had been treated by a departing resident. He had dutifully forewarned me that this patient had several stable medical problems and was on an archaic medical regimen that, contrary to good medical judgment, seemed to suit her just fine.

During our first visit together, I found Mrs Hines in good spirits, although she lamented the departure of her previous physician. "I had just broken him in," she informed me with a gleam in her eye. "You'll be around for awhile, won't you?" she questioned. I assured her that it was early in my residency, and I planned to continue in the clinic for at least another two or three years. She seemed satisfied with my reply, and then began to explore my personal life and background. "Are you married? Do you like Seattle? Do you live nearby?"

With some effort and diplomacy I refocused our discussion on her medical problems, noting anxiously that her systolic blood pressure was elevated to 194. I scanned her medical record and discovered that her blood pressure had been elevated during several previous clinic visits and that her medical regimen was woefully inadequate, with many of the prescribed doses being homeopathic. I explained to her the need to change her medications and promptly wrote a prescription for a potent, new antihypertensive agent. "Are you sure?" she appealed to me. "My last doctor always said I was doing so well."

I took her hand and reassured her, "I would feel uncomfortable not making a change at this time. The new blood pressure medicines are more effective and have fewer side effects than the older ones."

She smiled, picked up the prescription, and studied it intently. "I guess I can give it a try."

Of course I knew best. The potential consequences of long-standing hypertension, especially when poorly controlled, are myriad. But somehow, blinded by professional hubris, I had neglected to appreciate that Mrs Hines, without my assistance, had lived to be a spry octogenarian.

One day later, I realized the foible of that fateful encounter. As the medic-one doctor in the emergency room of a busy inner-city hospital, I was responsible for communicating with and supervising the area's paramedics. Late in the afternoon, I received a routine call. The medics were evaluating an 82-year-old woman who had fallen at home. She was complaining of severe dizziness and light-headedness when she attempted to sit up. Her pulse rate was 40 and her systolic blood pressure was 90. The paramedics wanted to bring her to a nearby private hospital for further evaluation and treatment. I agreed with their plan and asked for the name of her physician so I could notify that emergency room of her expected arrival. I then heard a high voice in the background in response to their inquiry: "Dr Gill is my doctor."

It couldn't be, but it was. That same voice that only yesterday had questioned, "Are you sure?" By now I was in a near panic. My pulse was 140. My head throbbed. My entire career flashed before my eyes. I thanked God I was already seated. Wiping the cold perspiration from my brow, I sheepishly completed my conversation with the medics and calmly (what self-control!) informed the private hospital to expect Mrs Hines in about 15 minutes, being careful not to divulge my true identity as the perpetrator of her medical crisis.

I was in a daze for the remainder of my ER shift, trying to convince myself that I was not responsible for this sudden mishap; but the temporal evidence was beyond dispute. My patient had been well. She saw me. I changed her medications. She was now in the hospital. All this had transpired within 24 hours. Guilty as charged!

Mrs Hines seemed happy to see me as I entered her hospital room the following morning. "That's my doctor," she pointed out proudly to the nurse who was taking her blood pressure. I asked her to explain what had happened. She stated that within one hour of taking the new medication she didn't feel well, experiencing "cold sweats" and a sensation of "seeing lights, like colored medallions." She must have noticed the look of remorse on my face, for she declared, "You mustn't blame yourself. I guess I'm just sensitive to new medicines. I've always been that way, you know." No, I didn't know. I hadn't taken the time to know.

Mrs Hines was discharged from the hospital after three days. Fortunately, she sustained no long-lasting ill effects from her hypotensive episode. For three years, I have followed her in my clinic, and her systolic blood pressure has remained elevated. She takes all of her previous medications at their former homeopathic but effective doses, and I have renewed this regimen on a quarterly basis. I saw her for the last time two weeks ago. We reminisced about our initial encounters together. I had just informed her that I would be leaving the clinic in two months, and that she would be reassigned to a new doctor. This time she took my hands in hers, perhaps perceiving my sense of loss and sadness. Several seconds passed in silence. Finally, her face brightened and she smiled. "I guess I'll have to break in another one."

Painful Lessons

Michael P. McCarthy, MD

> . . . He'll bring his charms to gladden you, and should his stay be brief,
> You'll have his lovely memories as solace for your grief.
>
> Edgar A. Guest, *To All Parents*

The central area of the pediatric station on which I worked was chronically underlit, and the resulting sense of gloom thus emitted seemed almost fitting, in a perverse sort of way. Of all the rotations taken that first year of family practice residency, none came close to matching pediatrics in terms of "depressogenesis." Although other rotations required longer hours, afforded less sleep, and produced more scut work, certain aspects of this one have cast a pall over my memory of Peds, now ten years in my past. But more than anything else, it was circumstances that forced me to confront my own weaknesses that now project the most persistent shadows.

In the rear-central area of the station stood a support pillar, and tacked onto it the poem "To All Parents." I struggled to convince myself that this poem was nothing more than maudlin hogwash and not even worth reading. Still, I found myself attracted to it, and when no one was looking I read it anyway. Always after reading its effort to explain a circumstance that defies explanation, that is, the death of a child, I felt foolish and embarrassed as I fought back the tears.

This pediatric rotation was held at a university hospital and as such catered mostly to seriously or chronically ill patients. All of the patients were the same age as my firstborn at that time. I felt I could show true sympathy toward these patients as I imagined my son with the different maladies seen in them. Likewise, I thought I was feeling true empathy for the parents of these patients when I saw them stumble around the ward as if in a blinding fog or somehow inebriated, their defense mechanisms working to numb them from what was happening to their children.

More than anything about general pediatrics, I remember Davy, a 17-month-old admitted with massive hepatosplenomegaly. After an exhaustive workup he had been given the diagnosis of reticuloendotheliosis with erythrophagocytosis. He was not responding to treatment, and his condition was rapidly deteriorating. In addition, he had developed a fever for which a cause was not immediately apparent. Broad-spectrum intravenous antibiotics were started while culture results were pending.

My team was not responsible for Davy's care, and I knew of him only from daily rounds with the other residents. One night, however, I came to know Davy in a way I will never forget.

This night came toward the end of my pediatrics rotation, and as first-year resident on call, I had been wakened to draw a gentamicin level from Davy. I had not been good at drawing blood from children, and, realizing Davy's extensive workup and treatment, I knew he would be an especially tough stick.

I walked into the treatment room where Davy, who had also been wakened, was waiting. I looked closely at him for the very first time and noted that his general emaciation, massive abdominal distension, and lesioned, mottled, and ecchymotic skin could not disguise what a truly handsome little boy he was, nor could they dim the wisdom that seemed to shine from his clear blue eyes.

I would routinely make three attempts at drawing blood before calling in my senior resident to do that which I could not. Routine was not followed this night as I lost track of the number of times I unsuccessfully pierced Davy. I justified my repeated attempts to the late hour and convinced myself that I was doing my senior resident a great favor by not waking him.

Again and again butterfly needles were stuck into scarred tissue, and lancets poked swollen heels. With each of my failed attempts Davy would moan weakly and gaze at me with tear-filled eyes. "Why are you hurting me?" they seemed to ask.

The nurse who was my assistant that night realized I would foolishly continue my efforts no matter how many times I failed. She witnessed Davy's pained, pleading eyes and heard his now barely audible moans. She wisely and mercifully suggested that perhaps the blood obtained from those multiple tries might be enough to run the ordered test. In so doing she provided a means of escape for this first-year resident who was too proud to admit defeat, as well as provided an excuse for this same resident who feared a possible angry reprisal from his senior resident, and who lacked ample moxie to waken him.

Two weeks after finishing my pediatrics rotation, I returned to the station to ask about Davy. I was saddened but not really surprised to learn he had died only a few days after I had left.

It's been said that some good comes from even the worst of experiences. I made many mistakes during this painful rotation, but I hope some lessons were learned.

I've always known that empathy and sympathy are both characteristic of a complete, well-rounded physician. I know now that, having never been in their situation, I really had no idea of the suffering and anguish felt by the parents of the patients on this pediatric ward. I realize now that empathy cannot be feigned, and the only person fooled was myself.

I did feel sorry for the patients with whom I dealt on this ward, but I also have seen firsthand how objectivity and professionalism can suffer when pity is mistaken for sympathy. Even basic procedures (like phlebotomies) may become difficult to perform as a result.

Finally, I hope I've learned never again to make a patient suffer because of my weaknesses. The pecking order of a hospital hierarchy and personal shortcomings, such as viewing authority figures with timidity and fear rather than seeing them as colleagues working toward the same end, should never hold precedence over a patient's care and comfort. Still the events of that night can never be rectified, and Davy and his questioning eyes remind me of this on a regular basis. Over the years, the questions asked have become more elaborate, more pointed:

"Why did you *keep* hurting me?"

"Why didn't you get somebody who knew what he or she was doing?"

"You knew I was dying, I knew I was dying. Was this particular blood test really necessary?"

"If it wasn't necessary, why did you make me suffer that much more on one of the last days of my brief life?"

After more than a decade, my totally unsatisfactory answer remains unchanged:

"Davy, I don't know."

Secondary Survey

Meg Verrees

Make sure your patient walks away smiling," the old surgeon opens the lunchtime skull session, the weekly conference that trails journal club. "Make sure a grin warms his face as he waves good-bye. See joy lighten his step when he turns to greet you. Ensure that your patient leaves happy. This is the most important lesson to learn in medicine." What is next most essential? one intern asks. Second in importance? a student in the group queries. The doctor speaking this afternoon is nearly deaf; most words seem to touch down then deflect from the pink shells of his ears. It takes three repeats for him to realize our prodding. As he considers the question, his voice falters for one moment, then from the lull comes out swinging. "The second most important skill to acquire in medicine," he calls out, "is vigilance. Vigilance!" He hesitates for a moment to allow this word time to settle. "Care, for example, in completing the secondary survey—that scouring with a clear eye, hardy ear, and sure hand of every curve and surface of a patient's skin."

The doctor plows onward: "In the hours flanking huge trauma, this careful sweep detects minor faults, slight injury. These points if missed later lead to distress. A good second look doesn't take skill. A complete follow-up check with a marauding eye and steady palm doesn't really even require intelligence. The healer in this instance simply needs vigilance." Silence once more follows this thought. Then the voice starts again. "Missing a small finding on the secondary survey will get you sued. Overt signs like a wound squirting blood or an open mouth gasping for breath won't get you in trouble. Everyone sees these big things and most realize the steps of proper treatment. And poor outcome emerging from the ash of wicked injury is always a fair possibility. But missing a subtle finding will trip you. Detecting covert signs through the waning haze of catastrophe separates the slick from the crude.

———————————

"Two medics wheel a patient from the landing pad outside the emergency department," the surgeon presents to the ring of six interns and students. "The man stretched on the gurney has just survived a plane crash that killed his three friends. You lift the sheet to discover that the cloth drapes a gash in his side that foams with each breath. Our man at rest appears thin save for a tight wedge of belly puffed beyond the clasp of his belt. A slash in his thigh spurts bright red blood. A bandage encircling the limb somewhat trims the flow. The lower leg points awkwardly toward a far corner of the trauma room. Against the metal side bar of the gurney his right arm lies crumpled and bent. And no matter how much you yell our man's name, he won't answer. Won't open his eyes. Won't turn and tell you to pipe down.

"So what do you do?" the doctor asks. "You fix him," the sage answers with ease. "These are all obvious signs. Injuries noted on the primary survey—that initial once-over with a coarse eye. No one misses these. Precisely where do you start? A tube slipped down his throat helps him breathe. A vent in his chest provides slick release for air escaping from the lung into the tight case of skin enclosing his chest. You repair the torn vessel in his belly and patch the snapped artery in his leg. You lift from the left side, from beneath the ladder of broken ribs, his ruptured spleen. You rejoin the leathery fragments of his torn bladder. You create for the shattered liver a safe place to heal. His arm and leg you straighten and bolt into place. And entry into the skull provides release of pooling blood. The long and wide tears in his skin you bathe and sew. All these you do in record time. Hooray for you!

"So the patient lives. But his days prove shaky for a while. The man stumbles. His constitution fails him. Old-time vice and true excess jump to the fore to cast rocks in his path. His are the tattooed, slow-healing lungs of a smoker. He proved not a meek drinker, so his stunned, sleepy liver lazily hands out blood clotting factors. Thus our man bleeds and bleeds. He ate a poor diet, so his skin mends slowly.

"But two months from the day of the accident, he strides from the hospital. He walks when two months before his legs couldn't bear weight. He holds a leather briefcase in each hand. Eight weeks before, his right arm refused to respond to command. He turns to briskly mull questions when on arrival he couldn't remember his name. He breathes easily; previously his lungs couldn't draw one wholesome breath. His skin glows warm and pink on that afternoon. Weeks before, as he passed through the swinging doors of the emergency department, he looked pale and felt chilled. His is a miraculous recovery. A wonderful cure. Cheers for our man. Hooray for you.

"But wait. As the man departs the grounds, a frown darkens his face. He scowls as he enters his car. One ripe glance reveals that the patient's right pinkie hangs twisted. The stubborn, small digit won't straighten or curl. Won't tuck or wriggle. The separate nubbin juts stiffly from the end of the man's working hand. It has fallen asleep. It is no longer one member of a vital family. It remains locked in place, an aloof guest at a table of chatty cousins.

"A true victor, our patient has reclaimed the life that was nigh wrenched away. He escaped the net death cast. That day he even looks hearty. But maybe fate has exacted a price to placate death. Or perhaps death has played a joke. Could be that death generously loosened its hold and granted one among us a short reprieve. More likely, beneath the hard crust of earth the sparse figure of death leans against the walls of its soiled den and grins. Our man has paid a price.

"The searching eye of one doctor stumbled. This faulty glance helped death collect its payment. The man has lost the use of one finger. Gone forever is a true player in his full set of ten. He rolls up his sleeves using nine. With four moving digits on his busiest hand he halts to wave hello to a friend. His nimble tenth digit has been replaced by a useless spare.

"The crisis over, on the secondary survey, a weak eye and shallow hand two months before missed two cracks in the bone of that finger. The caring eye of one doctor stumbled. And the man has paid for his life with one finger. He has lost the use of one petite, perky digit and been offered in its place one fleshy prong. A useless piece of skin mixed with bone. A frozen point. Part witch's crooked talon, part mummy's limp hook.

"Our man is angry. He's scowling. He's bitter.

"And he's a pianist."

A Father's Eyes

Stephen Schultz, MD

It is internship. Autumn. Shorter days, longer nights. I am doing pediatrics. It is 3:30 AM. I am answering a page to talk with parents on the infant floor. I have not yet been to bed, and my eyes have begun to burn. I want to lie down. I want to sleep. I enter the room. A young woman with long frizzy red hair sits just inside the door, facing away from me. She is rocking in a rocker, in short, clipped strokes that seem odd, almost frenetic. A man is sleeping on a cot, turned away from me. He is wearing Birkenstocks; the soles face me.

"Excuse me . . ." I trail off softly. It has been more than half an hour since I was called. I hope the question has answered itself. She looks up. I see now she's holding a baby.

"I'm Dr Schultz, the resident on call. Did you need to see me?"

"Oh, yes, Doctor. I'm glad you're here. I thought Daniel was looking a little bit more swollen, but I think he's better now. He's starting to breast-feed a little bit again, see there?"

I look down at a floppy, grotesquely swollen infant, perhaps 6 weeks old. He has a tube coming out of one nostril, and an IV in one hand. A nipple is being brushed across his lips as his mother persistently guides her breast to his mouth, but he is not making any movement at all. His eyes are swollen shut. My God, this kid looks bad. I am suddenly, painfully aware that in my haste to get to sleep, I have neglected to check the chart, or even to locate the name on the sign-out sheet to find out the principal diagnosis. What an idiot. A slow sensation of mild panic begins, similar to when I have to introduce someone whose name I should definitely know but cannot remember. This woman continues to talk, almost to herself. I am suddenly reminded of a crazy woman in *King of Hearts*, clutching a blanket she thinks is her baby. This kid is as interactive as a blanket.

Suddenly I know. This is the infant presented at morning report two days ago. Had a low-grade temp for two days, then spiked high. They took him to their doctor the third day, after he became lethargic. An LP was done. Sheets of polys, sheets of gram-positive cocci. Decreasing mental status. Transferred here. CT scan showed cerebral edema. NG tube placed secondary to inability to feed. Difficulty with fluid balance. Grim prognosis, unlikely to recover neurologically. Toasted squash.

"What do you think, Doctor?" I look down. Mom is looking up at me. I don't know what the question is. What am I doing here?

"What happened?" I turn around. Dad has woken up and is sitting on the edge of the bed. His hair is rumpled. He is hunched forward, his arms straight down at his sides, his hands clutching the sides of the cot.

I don't understand. "What?"

He straightens, looks up, and our eyes lock. "What happened?" he repeats softly, but more clearly.

I only have to look into those eyes for a second to know what he is asking. I realize he's not asking what happened to make this doctor come into this room at this hour. Three days later this man is still trying to sort out what happened to his son, what happened to the baby he already loved more fiercely than he thought it was possible to love. Will he live? Will he breast-feed again? Will he walk? Will he ever laugh with me? Oh, Sweet Jesus, please, what has happened to my son?

He looks away, and shakes his head. "I don't understand," he mumbles.

I stand in the center of the room. I don't know what to say, and very quickly I am unable to say anything. It is all I can do to suppress the ball of grief that is growing in my chest. Images of my own son fill my mind: the toothless grins and sweet breast-milk breath as a baby, the squeals of laughter of a mischievous toddler, the warmth of his sleeping body nestled in my protecting arms, the innocent questions that challenge me, make me pause, make me smile. The tricycle rides, the snowball fights, the ice cream cones, the love. And through it all, the fierce desire to protect him, to allow him to explore, but to shelter him from all harm. The love.

The rocker squeaks faintly, rhythmically.

Grief rises into my throat. "I . . . excuse me" is all I can say, and before I can even get out the door the tears start. I walk quickly past the nurses' station, and the sobs begin, like a vomiting spell that can be suppressed only so long, and once started cannot be controlled. A runner from transport walks by, staring. I duck into an unlit conference room, lean against the wall, and surrender to it, purge myself. It is the discordance of those father's eyes and the cynicism of "toasted squash," of sleep deprivation, of the insecurity of internship, of the fears of my own son's mortality. I cry for a long time.

My beeper goes off. I wipe my face, blow my nose. I don't go back into the room, and I don't leave a note.

I never see them again.

Hands On

Mark R. Fleisher, MD

The beeper flashes "2580." Rare is the house officer who relishes a call from the ICU. As I look for a phone, questions tumble through my mind. Is it about Bed 3 with the GI bleed? Has Bed 2 dropped his pressure again? I could have sworn that the woman in Bed 11 would have a quiet night on the vent. Maybe it's just my intern. I told her to call when she was hungry. I could use a snack too. How many pounds did I put on during this rotation? I pick up the phone across from Radiology as my beeper again flashes "2580." Someone's either really sick or really hungry.

"Hi. Did someone page me?"

"Bed 2 looks sick."

"I'm on my way."

It's amazing how a hospital evolves as it wades into the night. The aroma of microwaved popcorn and fried chicken hovers above the whirring floor-polishing machines. Dimmed hallways echo. The elevators move more quickly without the weight of roses and tiger lilies. Residents nod to each other as they pass.

Phone calls at 3 AM are not like other calls. They are passages. Choices must be made. Even if the decision is to do nothing at all, it is rarely effortless. Frost wrote of the road not taken. There are many roads to choose from on this snowy eve, especially in the ICU.

The door opens and the rite begins: soap, lather, rinse, dry, repeat, go to the bedside. The nurse was right: Bed 2 looks sick. Panting. Sweating. Moaning. Approaching the bed, I scan the monitor not for his vitals, but for his name. He has become Bed 2, the man with the stiff lungs and the stiffer heart. Bed 2 is the Blue Man. Next to him is the Yellow Man. People of color tend to inhabit the ICU.

"Mr West, what's wrong?"

"Call my wife." He grabs my hand and squeezes harder than his ventricle. "Call my wife." He's gurgling.

"Give him 100%. Where's the Lasix? Which one is the dobutamine? How high is the dopamine?" He is DNR. What are the limits?

Mr West rips off the face mask and wheezes, "Call my wife!"

Hopes rise as the wedge drops. I leave to call his wife. How do you wake someone at 3 AM? Does every phone call panic Mrs West? Surely she knows that Blue Men are not healthy. Does she take self-delusional solace that her husband is not the Yellow Man? I know what she is going to ask. I don't blame her. I would ask the same thing.

"Tell me, Doctor, should I come in?"

Suddenly, Bed 2 is no longer the Blue Man, no longer Bed 2 with the dreadful ejection fraction and the ghastly film. He is Mrs West's Mr West. Do I tell her to come in at 3 AM? How can I tell if this is his time? If he doesn't die tonight, will she believe me when I call her the next night? Am I being an alarmist? Choices have to be made.

"He's asking for you. You should come in."

She must dress, and then call her son to drive her to the hospital. The only traffic at 3 AM is delivery trucks and distraught families. How do you get dressed knowing your husband is dying and asking for you? Do you consciously choose which clothes to wear? What have I done to her?

Mr West is panting. He's motioning for me.

"Did you call her?"

"Yes, she's on her way."

"Good," and he closes his eyes as I open the drips wide. His breathing quickens and his numbers deteriorate. I check and recheck the jumble of lines. What else could I add? What should I subtract? Looking at Mr West, I am ashamed of how I abetted in stripping him of his essence, of himself. It started, I know, with the hospital gown's voyeuristic rearlessness. I never knocked on his door. I referred to him as a case, a bed, a color. Looking at Mr West, all I want to do is keep him alive. What am I forgetting?

Mr West knows. With his eyes closed and his mouth agape, he takes my hand. I am still. We hold hands. He doesn't improve but he doesn't worsen. Twenty minutes later, his wife and son arrive. They look at our interlocked fingers and understand. I give his hand to her and leave the room. She knows.

Regaining Compassion

James W. Lynch, Jr, MD

Rounds were over—finally—and I was exhausted. I kept reminding myself that every July is the same. The new interns and students were both petrified and striving to make a good impression, which translated into long and sometimes painful bedside rounds.

There was, however, a bright spot, and her name was Kelli. A third-year student assigned to our oncology service as her first rotation, Kelli offered refreshing enthusiasm, charm, and encouragement daily to her patients. But today something was different. She came to me and asked for a few minutes to talk behind closed doors. Almost immediately she began to weep and between sobs she laid her heart before me: "I feel so inadequate. The *only* thing I have to offer is my compassion. But now I wonder what my words can mean as I look at Sheila. It's all so overwhelming. I'm not sure I can keep doing this."

Sheila was the 35-year-old mother of four, all younger than 12, whose husband, Michael, worked as a nurse at our hospital. After a brief bout with "walking pneumonia" that didn't resolve, she was diagnosed with metastatic non–small cell lung cancer and had been admitted for chemotherapy. Her chief complaint was an enlarging mass, a finding whose significance had escaped neither Sheila nor Kelli. The gentle but honest conversation mixing tears, facts, faith, and human touch had been all Kelli (and I) could bear. I had already given my sermon to the students about the profound sense of peace and joy our patients often find through their suffering, and at the time my talk was well received. But now Kelli's eyes begged for more than a philosophy lecture or a pat on the back. So I prayed for both of us to be given the wisdom and strength to give the best care to Sheila, after which Kelli smiled, wiped her eyes, and returned to her work.

During that month Kelli had several opportunities to practice her "only" contribution to Sheila's care. Sheila was able to share with her the full range of emotions common to all who have struggled with cancer: fear of death, anger with the unfairness of it all, sadness at the prospect of her children growing up with no mother, joy at small successes in the day-to-day struggle, and gratitude for our efforts. "My pain is much better today. Thanks for all you're doing for me." Finally, she was able to go home—as it turned out, for the last time.

Kelli continued to work hard learning medicine and punctuating rounds with her kindness and humor. All of her patients adored her, especially one in particular, Mr Bernard. He was admitted with one of his many exacerbations of bronchiectasis and was receiving traditional medical treatment with inhalational therapy and parenteral antibiotics. Quite unexpectedly one day, however, his cough worsened and respiratory distress rapidly led to the need for mechanical ventilation. Here again, Kelli brought her special skill to the bedside. As the anesthesiologist gained control of the patient's airway via nasotracheal intubation, Kelli sat at the bedside and, recognizing the terror on Mr Bernard's face, began stroking his hand and explaining every step of the procedure. "Now, Mr Bernard, I know this tube is uncomfortable, but we need it to help you breathe. Hold my hand. I'll stay with you." His viselike grip on her warm hand was all the evidence I needed that he had heard and appreciated her. She accompanied him to the intensive care unit, where Michael was at work setting up the ventilator and preparing for yet another patient who had "crashed."

Our ICU, like most, is staffed by superb nurses, and Sheila's husband Michael was widely regarded as one of the most skilled. Kelli remained with Mr Bernard until he was sufficiently stable and then came back to our workroom. She then asked, "What should I have done differently? Why did he get so sick? Were we using the wrong antibiotic or bronchodilator?" As a team of students, interns, and resident, we reviewed the medical facts surrounding the case and concluded that no other medical intervention would have prevented the ICU transfer. While we were talking, there was a knock on the door. Michael's head and upper body emerged as he peered into the room. He looked shaken, staring at the floor as he removed his glasses and rubbed his eyes. Fearing the worst I asked, "Is Sheila all right?" He just nodded and for what seemed a long time said nothing.

Certain moments seem to take on a life of their own: Some joyful, others painful, and still others an odd combination of both, but all living on because of a rare connection with both the mind and the heart. Michael began, "I just wanted to tell you, all of you, how much Sheila and I appreciate the care she's getting. It's not just the medical stuff, I mean, that's important and we know she's getting the best medical treatment available. But it's the way you *take care* of her"—he paused—"and me that makes it so different." He pressed his thumb and index finger into his tearing eyes and stopped to regain his composure. Everyone was silent as we tried to hold back our own tears and listen to the rest of his message. He then looked at Kelli and said, "Kelli, I was watching you hold that man's hand. I listened as you talked to him and I tell you, do you know how long it's been since I held anyone's hand in there, or thought about how it must feel to be on one of those things?" We still said nothing as he again began to cry. "I want you to know, Kelli, that you, and each of you, have reminded me about something I had long forgotten in my job. And I won't forget again to comfort those I take care of. Thank you all." With this he entered the room and after warmly embracing each of us he slipped out, leaving a room full of blurry-eyed physicians.

Everyone sat motionless and silent for a minute or two, trying to absorb the impact of what had just transpired. Eventually we all returned to caring for our patients, but none of us will ever forget the intense sense of joy and sorrow mingled in that room.

It has been almost two years since that day and now Kelli is the mother of a beautiful 2-week-old boy and awaiting graduation next month. Recently, as Kelli and I were chatting about motherhood, our discussion turned to Sheila and Michael. Looking back, she continues to underestimate her "medical" contributions to her patients' care while being grateful for the opportunity to comfort them. But as she is ready to graduate, feeling more confident in her skills as a physician, she remembers the profound hope and purpose she found. And she reminds me that "Among all the things we do, what our patients are most likely to remember is our compassion."

Watchers

L. Stewart Massad, MD

Stay and watch," she'd said.

A thin hand on a thin blanket. A twist of IV tubing on a sheet. A closed door, black windows, faded gown. The rasp of agonal breathing wears through a doctor's defenses, into his heart.

"Stay and watch," she'd once said.

A decade and more ago, in another life, I was an intern. On the obstetrics service, I was a hotshot: thought I was better than I was, and I was better than most. Efficient, hard, angry, and young, after four years in medical school I'd memorized figures and physiology, tables, drug doses, and arrogance.

Then, too, there'd been a twist of IV tubing on a hospital sheet, and blackness in other windows, but on that night my patient's hard breathing was the herald not of death but of life. She was a 17-year-old mother of two on her way to becoming a mother of three. It was a slow night, and I had nothing else to do but sleep. Still, I took her history, calculated her gestational age, finished her physical, drew her blood, and glanced at her monitor strip in under 15 minutes. I nodded to her, wished her the best, and headed for the door promising to be back for the baby's birth.

"Stay and watch," her nurse had said.

Leah sat between windows, arms folded under a wise woman's frown. I gaped, trying to think of an answer. But my training had taught me how to give orders to nurses, not how to talk to them.

She nodded at the admission note on my clipboard.

"Learn anything from that?" she asked.

I looked at two pages of scribble, the summary of a pregnant woman's normality, and shrugged.

"But I thought you boys were here to learn," she taunted. Her lips smiled but not her eyes, and her smile was a challenge, as loud in that room as derisive laughter. When I did not storm out, she softened. "Stay and watch," she offered again. "See what it takes for a woman to bring a child into this world."

I was too young to walk away from a dare. We watched as the baby came down, careless of its mother's cries. We delivered the child in the labor room with the father looking on. That was Leah's idea—heresy in those days—but all the senior residents were asleep, all the attendings still at home.

Over four years, Leah taught me to be an obstetrician. More, she taught me to be a physician, taught me to see, to feel, to listen, to touch, to speak, to understand. She showed me what she—or I, or anyone with compassion and time—could do to ease the troubles of childbirth. Leah taught me to sense labor's slow cadences: the three-minute beat of contractions, the crescendo of pants and grunts and moans that ended with an infant's cry. She taught me to read the trajectory of a child's descent in the way a woman twisted, to see which would go bad, which would end with the knife. She taught me to talk down screaming children birthing children, to massage away the ache of back labor, to coach women into puffing their fears away.

"Stay and watch," she'd said.

But I was a surgeon at heart and would not stay long. From the upstate hospital I went down to the city and an oncology fellowship. There I learned to forget Leah's lessons: cancer, like the sun, blinds those who look on too directly.

I was gone eight years. I came back to head a division at the university where I had trained. No one from my resident class had stayed. The junior faculty who'd taught us had grown gray. The old chairman had been forced out. My favorite mentor had retired. There was a rumor that Leah had set up as a nurse midwife in a small town nearby. Passing through once on the community hospitals' grand rounds circuit, I tried to track her down, but if she'd been there, she'd moved on and left no memories.

It was Leah who found me, finally. She came to my office, self-referred, with a folder full of photocopies and a plastic box of slides: neuroendocrine carcinoma of the cervix. She had lost weight but not heart, had cut her hair but kept her smile. We chatted about our pasts, our plans, and disappointments. We talked about her future, both knowing she had none. It was a quiet meeting, except for the thumping of my heart.

Radical surgery, chemotherapy, radiation: she'd endured all, knowing their futility. Always a professional, she watched herself die and reported to me every symptom of her slow decline: the site and radiation of her pain, the crackling of her skin, the frequency of stools and vomitus, her tremor, her stoop, her hobble, her cough.

"Stay and watch," she'd said, so long ago.

We were through with that now. Eleven days ago a brain metastasis had bled. Her kidneys had failed soon after. Her lungs were choked with cancer. Riddled too with tumor, her liver was dying. Her heart, so steady for so long, bucked and fluttered.

The humor and the light, the wisdom and the joy of her all were gone. I should have been gone too, should have gone home hours before: I had surgery and a full afternoon's clinic ahead, and nothing to offer Leah but saline, morphine, and oxygen. I knew she would not live to thank me. Still, I stayed. I watched.

I watched her breath suck in and out inside the mask. Her half-lidded eyes fluttered with the effort. Just before dawn, she quit.

A penlight in her eyes, two fingers at her throat, a stethoscope on the washboard of her ribs, and it was over. I might have said good-bye, but the woman who would have heard had gone.

Outside, I leaned against the cool brick of the hospital, facing east, where a red sun rose over a new world. I was tired. I wanted to go home and rest, longed to sit and sip coffee and listen to birds wake. But I had debts to the dead that I could pay only to the living.

"Stay and watch," she'd said. I did.

A Vacation Fit for a Собака

Nancy L. Greengold, MD

When my vacation time approached this year, I wallowed in my glorious options. I pored over the European hot spots in the newspaper's travel section, and then remembered I hated to fly. I thought about taking the "drive up the coast," then parked the idea, recalling my last boilover on the Grapevine. I imagined fleetingly the joy of doing nothing for two weeks, but felt uneasily self-indulgent. When the responsibility of "having a vacation" began to weigh on me, I decided my dream of a California tan would have to fade. I was going to spend eight hours each day learning Russian, a language that was barbed wire to my ears.

Before I reached this decision, the Russian language had had nothing but negative connotations for me. I had spent the first two years of residency "taking care" of Russian-speaking clinic patients who could not understand a word I said. My every interview and examination of them was under the constant supervision of one of several translators, who censored our conversations and usurped all of my medical authority. Rarely did I achieve eye contact: the patient's attention was always bestowed entirely on my nemesis and life preserver, the translator.

I had become a mere fly in the medical ointment, buzzing historical questions that I hoped were being properly translated. The translator would swat me down from time to time: "We don't say things like that. You can't tell him he has cancer. It will depress him for no reason." I would listen to the violent foreign words that assaulted my ears. I would ask a simple question, the translator would mutter something in Russian, and the patient's answer would come back thick as a lawyer's summation. Translation: "She says not good. Her stomach hurts, but I can tell you, she's a complainer." Often the translator would tell me in the patient's presence: "These people! They do not take their medicines except when they feel bad. They do not listen to you. You are wasting your time trying to get through to them."

Occasionally, battles would be waged between the patient and the enraged translator, who would lapse into outright verbal abuse. The translator would then turn to me, exasperated, saying, "These people! They go out and see other doctors and get their favorite medicines. I told this man that if he does this again, he will be kicked out of the clinic." She expected my thanks.

In fact, the translators could not comprehend ungrateful young doctors like me. They did their best to simplify our jobs by "anticipating" our routine questions, asking patients about cardiac risk factors even before we did, and giving out free advice and medical information they "figured" we would want to give.

It was torture. I experienced the Pavlovian rush of nausea when 1 PM approached each Thursday, which signaled clinic.

So did my colleagues. With no real direct communication with our patients, we felt as if we were practicing veterinary medicine. We griped and groaned when the clinic afternoon arrived, and we knew the Russians were coming. *Oy vay*, we would lament. The one and only Russian word we knew was *baleet* ("pain"). All we heard from the Russians was *baleet, baleet, baleet*. We came to hate our patients. We came to hate ourselves.

Could my short vacation be used to traverse the barrier that stood between me and my patients? Could I come to see them as more than just dumb animals, barking their needs at me?

On the first day of my language tutorial, I was introduced to Nanka, the Bulgarian professor who was to teach me Russian. Nanka never said a word in English. She bombarded me with foreign words. She talked, she coaxed, she shouted at me, pointing to this and to that, playing Annie Sullivan to my Helen Keller; I could neither hear nor see what she was driving at.

She taught me the terms for everything in the room: the table, the chair, the floor. When I finally named everything successfully, she switched to prepositions and I was lost again. My agreements didn't make sense. I could not grasp the genitive, the accusative, the dative. Why, I wondered, did someone design such a foolish language? Why use multisyllabic words for such simple things? Why connect words with consonants that force you to spit? I complained but my teacher ignored me: She kept talking, cajoling, hammering at me.

Was this my just dessert? Had I yacked this way at the Russians in clinic? Had I been totally unaware of their feelings when I unceremoniously told them to take off all of their clothes (layers and layers of them!) so that I could proceed with my examination? Here, even fully dressed, I felt completely exposed: stupid, ignorant, alien.

For two weeks I was like a dog, living for the occasional smile of my teacher, for the rare pat on the back, the words of encouragement when I did something well; one day, she brought me *hlep* ("bread") after I did a lesson particularly well, and I wolfed it down happily. I suffered bitterly when she disapproved of my homework and insinuated that I did not follow her instructions correctly. Had I frowned similarly at patients because they told me they took their medicine but the blood pressures belied the fact?

While I questioned myself, I persevered, struggling through the jungle of words with my machete of blind faith. I asked my teacher to help me develop a medicine-specific vocabulary. She rallied to the cause, forcing her delicate mouth to give me the words for *mucous, diarrhea*, and *vomit*. While most students sought sentences for "Where is the train station?" I wanted her to craft, "Have you had any discharge from your penis?"

During my two weeks of study, I learned a little Russian. More than that, I discovered how it felt to be infantilized, to have fallen from professional grace because of language deficiency. I learned firsthand what I had been doing to my patients for the past two years.

I am now back at work in my R3 year, practicing medicine, diligently stumbling along in the morass of medical/conversational Russian. Thursday afternoon clinic is no longer intolerable. I can be a physician.

In fact, I am incredibly conspicuous now. The translators find me cute. They encourage my interaction with patients, now assuming the role of editors; they no longer seize the helm of conversations when I ask for help, out of either respect for me or fear that I understand. They are generous in their praise. My grammar may be a little cockeyed, but they relish my enthusiasm for their language, my growing love of their culture. I am an honorary Russian!

And the patients? They too claim to be charmed by my efforts. They look at me now and more than a few who formerly were mute have miraculously begun attempting to speak English in response to my baby steps toward them in Russian. Often the patients forget their multiple chief complaints in favor of discussing The Motherland, in favor of becoming my teacher. And, I must admit, at times it seems that my patients patronize me just a wee bit. They smile at my funny mis-conjugations and dys-declensions. And, of course, before they leave me and in our Russian manner, they grab my silly face and kiss both cheeks.

I am indebted to Mark Ault, MD, and the Department of Medicine at Cedars-Sinai Medical Center for their support of and enthusiasm for my endeavor to communicate more effectively with my patients.—N.L.G.

Собака *is the Russian word for* dog.—ED.

The Person *With* the Disease

Clifton K. Meador, MD

The hospital where I trained during my residency had one of the early diabetic-metabolic units. Whenever a patient with diabetic acidosis was admitted, the entire medical service mobilized. We followed many bio-chemically driven rituals and protocols. I forget how many consecutive patients we had without a death, but it must have been near the world's record at that time. If there was any disease I was ready for, it was the treatment of patients with complex diabetes. At least that's what I believed before I was drafted into the Army Medical Corps and met Amy.

For several months before I took over her care, 11-year-old Amy's diabetic control had become extremely brittle. She could progress from the unconsciousness of severe hypoglycemia in early morning to coma due to diabetic ketoacidosis by bedtime and vice versa. And she had been experiencing this with increasing frequency. Because of the other mundane demands on my time at the army post where I was serving, I was exhilarated to take on this complicated clinical challenge. I was certain I could correct the situation in little time.

I did not know how wrong I would turn out to be.

No matter what I tried, nothing worked. I changed Amy's diet a dozen different ways. I switched from one type of insulin to another. I split the doses into all kinds of combinations. I started her on regular insulin before each meal and at bedtime. I cut her insulin dose drastically, hoping to reduce rebound hyperglycemia. Despite all my efforts, she continued the pattern of erratic swings of blood sugars.

Within several months I thought I had considered every possible contributing factor for her brittle state. I had her seen by several local consultants. Nothing changed. I tried to refer her to a prominent clinic or to Walter Reed Hospital. The family refused. I was devoting a large amount of my time to the care of this one patient. Every plan I tried either made her condition worse or had no effect on stabilizing her blood glucose levels. I was stuck with Amy and she with me.

Then Amy and her mother disappeared. At first I was relieved, but I began to wonder and then worry. None of the other medical officers had seen her, so I assumed she had gone into the civilian medical community or to one of the major clinics.

I did not see Amy again for more than four months. One day she and her mother appeared in the waiting room of the dispensary. I was apprehensive when I saw them. However, both were smiling and moved toward me rapidly. Both were talking at the same time. At first, I could not make out what they were telling me. Finally the mother spoke alone. She told me that Amy had not had a hypoglycemic episode or been acidotic in more than three months. Most of her urine tests for sugar and acetone were negative. (This was in the days before fingerstick blood glucose monitoring.)

I could not wait to hear how they had achieved such a striking turnaround. What had I failed to do? What combination of insulin and diet was she following? Was she taking some new drug I had not heard of? What physician had been able to do what I could not? My curiosity was wild. How had they corrected this biochemical and physiological dilemma?

"How do you account for this remarkable change?" I finally asked.

The mother shook her head in puzzlement and, extending her hands palms up, shrugged her shoulders. "All we know is several things happened about the same time." She went on to tell the story of a new family moving in across the street four months ago. They had a 3-year-old daughter. Amy had become the child's babysitter on an almost daily basis. Also, about the same time, the mother and father had given Amy a kitten. Concomitant with the babysitting and caring for the kitten, the wild swings in blood sugars ceased within a week. Amy and her mother laughed as they told me the story. I was bewildered. I made a few inane comments, and then they left.

At the time I felt defeated. I just could not accept the relation of Amy's smoothed clinical course to something as preposterous as a kitten and babysitting. I continued to search for biochemical explanations. Maybe, unbeknownst to me, her mother had been doing something strange with Amy's diet and stopped it. Perhaps she started following her diet or she took her insulin like it was prescribed. I knew that none of these explanations answered my questions. As I had been trained, I had watched Amy by the bedside in the hospital and had seen the wild biochemical oscillations occur under the closest observations. Finally I simply had to admit that manipulating only the variables of diet, fluids, and insulin had failed. Yet some factor related to a small kitten and a young child had succeeded. I continued to see Amy and her mother every two or three months after that episode. Amy continued to do well until I left the Army more than a year later.

I have thought about Amy many times over the years. I now know that she taught me volumes: to look for those things we cannot measure in a test tube; to know that the manifestations of disease are often the result of strange combinations, and interactions of people, moods, beliefs, objects, and places do affect our physiology and biochemistry; to realize that the severity and course of a disease is sometimes unique to the life events of a single patient.

I learned that uncovering these individualized ameliorating and aggravating factors can be quite a challenge. I found that I could assist patients in searching for these peculiar influences by asking them two unspecified questions: What are you doing in your life that you should not be doing? What should you be doing in your life that you are not? Using this gentle, probing approach, I have encountered other patients with unexpected elements in their lives: diabetic acidosis precipitated by the unwanted visit of an irritating daughter-in-law on Christmas Eve; severe diarrhea associated with an embezzling and threatening boss; recurring severe headaches in the mother of an oversolicitous unmarried daughter; dizzy spells induced by the profanity of the driving partner of a fundamentally religious truck driver; and, in a most fascinating patient, abdominal cramps and diarrhea associated with a specific brand of toothpaste. All of these patients improved when the life factors were confronted or eliminated.

So Amy initiated the expansion of my narrow model of disease, which had been far too constricted into the abstractions of chemistry and physics. My experience with her reaffirmed the truth of the old statement: It is as important to know the person *with* the disease as it is to know the disease. To this we should remind ourselves and add: It is equally important to know about the people, the places, the things, the beliefs . . . even the small animals that surround the person with the disease. Amy was the first to teach me that nothing clinical occurs in isolation.

Holding the Heart

Daniel J. Waters, DO

It is something I take for granted, now. Something I have assistants to do. But to hold the living heart of another human being is among the rarest of privileges. Those so favored should never lose sight of the inherent mystery and wonder of the experience. When you hold the heart you can know its story. You can read, as if in Braille, the brittle threads of atherosclerosis. You can feel the heft of ventricular hypertrophy or the flaccid ennui of dilated cardiomyopathy. When you hold the heart you can know *almost* all of its secrets.

Today's cardiac operations are dazzling exercises in manometrics and surgical technics. Meters of catheters and miles of coaxial cable that terminate in screens glowing with iridescent numbers and waveforms. Endless streams of shifting parameters—but all of it is exposition, none of it plot. These stories are truly writ in blood. And you can only read them with your hands. Open the cover that is the sternum. Turn back the frontispiece of the pericardium. Take a moment to watch the contractions—the foreword for this story. Run a gloved finger over the surface, like over the lines of a page. With your palm make a gentle cradle for this weighty volume. Here is the leathery scar of an old infarction. There, the hydraulic thrill from a regurgitant valve. Some hearts are so petrified with calcium that you must lift them gingerly, almost tenderly, for fear they might actually break.

When it is unsupported by the pump-oxygenator, we approach the heart like a bashful suitor. A gentle caress of the chambers or a delicate draw on the epicardium is all we are permitted. The heart is in control and here we are mindful of its power and its petulance, its disdain for outside agitation. But once it is "on the pump"—cross-clamped—we turn brutish. This resolute organ, which had not known pause in its cycle for decades, lies pale and motionless—a study in diastolic defeat. Now we grope and manipulate with abandon. Bending, twisting, folding the muscle in constant pursuit of better exposure. Frigid and paralyzed, the heart does not resist our advances. We do what we must and try to finish quickly, for we know this can be but a brief interlude. With each passing minute we test the limit of the heart's endurance, its capacity for forgiveness. Done with our assault, we release the steel stranglehold. Warmed blood flows, washing out the occupying army of potassium ions like Pharaoh's chariots at the Red Sea. The millivolt gradient on which life depends is restored. The heart stirs.

Some hearts awaken as if refreshed by a midday nap, ready to return to the work at hand. Others struggle to regain their lost vigor, stunned by a monstrous anoxic hangover. A few stutter in the panic of fibrillation, awaiting salvation by the lightning bolt of cardioversion. The heart-lung machine, its thirst for venous return slaked, now yields back its treasure of cells and plasma. Chambers fill. Gossamer leaflets flutter. The intrusive cannulas are banished and their rents drawn closed with silken purse strings. Invisible leaks miraculously seal. Attention turns from the story to the book, for the ink must be dry before we dare close the cover.

"The heart," said William Harvey, "is a pump." Once and again.

My medical colleagues have told me that it is angiography that tells the real story of heart disease. Like Plato's cave dwellers, they see shadows and assume them substance. Bland, dichromatic, two-dimensional. Like beholding the Sistine Chapel through the eyepiece of a video camera. Many see the disease. Fewer understand it. Only the surgeon, I believe, truly comes to know it. "Don't you get tired of doing the same thing over and over?" they ask. As if any story like this could be the same as the one before. Pulling taut the wires as I close the incision, I know how the Sultan must have felt.

Tell me another story.

Tell me again.

Beginnings

Carolyn Wolf-Gould, MD

It is now 16 hours before the first patient is due to arrive at our new practice, and I am at the office searching for a Band-Aid for the blister on my heel. Even as I rummage through the cardboard cartons strewn about the floor, I know that the chances of my actually finding one here are remote. We have no desks, no immunizations, no guaiac cards, no charts, no computer, no . . . but why focus on the things we do not have? What we do have is far more important: four family physicians straight from residency wringing their hands, a motivated staff of five milling around in directionless circles, and a lovely office with beautifully painted walls and shiny new examination tables. Desks? Who needs desks when we can sit on the new carpet? Toilets? Who needs toilets when patients can easily use the facilities at the YMCA across the street? Another thing we do have is flowers. Lots of them: fall bouquets of daisy and Queen Anne's lace from our parents, an orchid from an orthopedic surgeon, and an orange tree from an obstetrician. There are faded plastic flowers scattered on the furniture in the waiting room, and no one seems to know where they came from. A potted ivy sits on the temporary counter in the unfinished nursing station on the exact spot where the computer was supposed to go, had it arrived. My husband, Chris, says plants are more aesthetic than computers anyway, more healing, so we are glad that it is there. Oh yes, I forgot the fish tank. We have a fish tank, too. No fish, but there is a plastic sunken battleship and an attachment for making bubbles. We also have an abundance of fruit flies. They have resisted our office manager's attempts at spraying and spring from the sink in joyous clouds whenever we run the tap.

This isn't how I imagined it would be to start practice, but much of life unfolds in ways I do not expect. I did not expect I would marry the bearded man who worked on the adjacent cadaver in anatomy class. But here we are, not only married but job-sharing so that we are able to care for our son. I did not expect that Carl and Jennifer would decide to job-share and agree to move to this small town to practice with us. But there they are, sitting on the floor in our deskless office worrying about the fruit flies. Our respective toddlers, Jesse and Olivia, are oblivious to the careful plans we four have made to create time and space in our lives to care for them. They are here with us today, chasing each other around the empty rooms and opening the drawers to the exam tables.

Chris sees the first patient tomorrow. On the schedule it says, "Rule out sexually transmitted disease." We have checked. There is no chocolate agar, no chlamydia culture, and no HIV consent form. Chris says he's going to "wing it," whatever that means. I just hope he doesn't get arrested.

We hang our diplomas on the wall to remind us that we finished high school, college, medical school, and residency and even passed the boards. The fruit flies land on the frames in random punctuation. All our years of training for this, for tomorrow. We are hopeful that there will be Band-Aids in the office when the patients arrive in the morning. We order pizza, sit on the new carpet with toddlers on our laps, and plan for the kind of health care we hope to provide. Jennifer writes *Vision* at the top of a sheet of white paper and we create a list: access to all, community-oriented primary care, family systems approach to medicine. As the list grows our spirits rise. We know that we are green and idealistic and revel in this moment when we feel we can accomplish it all.

In the fish tank a stream of white bubbles rises from the bottom of the tank to burst at the surface. Jesse and Olivia are enthralled. We four parents/doctors watch the fruit flies settle on the pizza crusts and know that the joys and worries of this day will soon be replaced by the larger task of caring for patients in this small town. We know it will be a struggle to maintain a balance between the needs of our practice and those of our children. We have a sense that we are breaking new ground with our double job-share, double-parenting strategy, and we wonder who we will look to for guidance. We wonder if we can pull it off. The moment of green idealism has passed, and the reality of being new attendings in a new place looms enormous and gray. We get up and resume our search through cardboard boxes for chocolate agar, Band-Aids, and immunizations. There is much to accomplish before our practice resembles the list we have just created. We roll up our sleeves and continue to work. Jesse and Olivia help.

The Reward

L. Stewart Massad, MD

Through fog, headlight beams pick out only gray road and white lines. Like seconds off a clock, like moments from a life expended driving from home to hospital, hospital to home, those lines tick by. Half-hidden trees, bridges, houses hover on the edge of vision like memories of old mistakes. I would linger and look, linger and dream, but . . .

At the hospital, a woman labors: her third child, and I must hurry. I struggle to recall her history, my mind still charged with sleep. I still feel cotton sheets and woolen blankets and the grumpy woman wakened out of time yet who rouses herself to say good-bye to me (the taste of her skin, the scent of her kiss). I still hear my 12-year-old call "Daddy?" as I slip past the room at the head of the stairs, leaving behind only promises, only promises.

I find myself on the labor suite with fingers at my patient's cervix and no recollection of the journey there: the years tell, and I am growing old. The baby's head is deep in the pelvis, right occiput anterior, with little molding. We—mother, father, daughter, doctor—will not wait long.

I run the monitor tracing through my fingers like a stockbroker trying to read the value of life off a ticker tape, like a telegraphist trying to decode the future of the world. I shake my head: absurd—the baby's fine; that's all an obstetrician needs to know.

The woman and her husband look to me for reassurance. I give it. It's cheap enough after all, though they treasure it, though I've withheld it too many times to recall, on wild rides to the section room. I speak to the nurse, then wander into the hall.

The ward is full of the thump of fetal heartbeats, 120 to 160 cycles per minute, magnified and amplified. Those are the drumbeats of an untamed generation come to take my place in the world. They can have it. I feel my age, want only to be home.

I stop at the nursing station for coffee and a joke. The coffee is bitter, the joke stale. But we drink and laugh: tired ourselves, we forgive each other our tiresomeness.

Changed into scrubs, I stand by the labor board and wait. The names on the wall mean nothing. Only lists of cervical diameters, graphs of dilation and descent, catalogues of complications signify. My mind drifts.

Then the animal cry of bearing down comes from my patient's room. A rush of adrenaline clears my brain. I recall the beautiful woman distended with child and the handsome young man beside her. I mask and gown and glove, then stand by doing nothing—well, I elevate the chin a bit, to spare the soft parts, but the mother does the work.

The shoulders stick. The face between the woman's legs works like a landed fish. I reach inside the birth canal, turn the baby, free an arm. That's all it is: a simple thing, to save a life. In a gush of fluid the newborn spills out.

The father whoops, the mother falls back on the table pad. The child is pink as a prom carnation, a girl. She kicks, twists, beats her little fists against my hands. I reach for a towel and dry her, rubbing with the rough cloth until her skin glows. I swaddle her in green hospital cotton. Ready to clamp the cord, I cradle her against my body, and then, like the morning that is breaking through the hospital windows,

she opens her eyes.

Identity Matters (or Does It?)

Zira DeFries, MD

Any number of people have asked me how it feels to be retired. Sometimes I say it feels great, other times I say it's OK, but mostly I say ask me next year. After 54 years of practicing medicine, of using the doctor insignia fore and aft my name, of being immersed in a tightly woven medical belief system, reinforced daily by a busy psychiatric practice, I had little time to ponder the significance implicit in a heretofore uncritically assumed doctor identity (DI). It was a given—helping patients fashion *their* identity took precedence. I took mine for granted—ie, until the day of reckoning came 'round, the day I'd set to retire, the day I was unceremoniously transformed from a "professional" to a "civilian."

Although I had long since shed that unassailable doctor symbol, the white coat, I now felt truly defrocked, naked, without even so much as a fledgling postdoc identity on the horizon. The urge to fashion a successor, one better attuned to my impending status, took hold with a vengeance. For starters, I marshaled in my mind the many rewards of retirement: no more malpractice insurance premiums to pay; I could scale down the number of journal subscriptions and medical societies I'd felt obliged to join to stay on the cutting edge; a reprieve from attending CME courses invariably given at the most inconvenient times and locations. I could trash with complete impunity the innumerable bureaucratic proclamations handed down from on high by the corporate sentinels of managed care; I could bask in the newfound freedom of not having to keep meticulous history and progress notes for the express purpose of warding off the malpractice police. The ne plus ultra, though, was deliverance from the worry about patients whose self-destructive behavior was out of my control but for whom I nonetheless felt responsible.

Exulting in these newfound exculpations was, however, tempered by the still-vivid memory of the trauma of dismantling my office. Disposing of unused batches of prescription pads, triplicates, stationery, Kleenex, couch, clock, and other appurtenances essential for a respectable New York City psychiatrist's office was wearisome enough, but relocating the mountainous pile of accumulated case records—which had over the years been carefully guarded on the outside chance in the distant future some lawyer, somewhere, might demand validations of his grown client's deranged mind when that client was a child: at that point I rued the day I had opted to retire.

Now with an empty office, gaping hourly slots in my appointment book, all usual practice chores irrelevant, I was left with an empty agenda, giving me ample time to muse about my newly acquired limbolike state. Who am I anyway, without the doctor regalia and paraphernalia that had nourished me for more than half a century, that had led me to believe my DI would never waiver, was immutable? The undeviating path I trod over the years when I woke at 7, headed for my office at 8, saw my first patient at 9, followed by the next at 10, and so on till the end of the day, when days turned to weeks, weeks to months, months to years, until one artificially chosen day the routine came to a halt, the solid structure, the calendar markers gone. Patients' problems no longer took precedence over my own. Time took on an unfamiliar face, loomed endless at the same time I was conscious of how finite time had suddenly become. The invisible plumb line that united the fragments and diverse facets of my life became startlingly real, almost palpable, thwarting any dreams of a rose-colored future yet to come. A voice within said: You had better build a noetic scaffolding to cling to as you wend your way through shrinking time.

So back to the sempiternal question: Who the devil am I now that I'm retired? Do I hang on to the original DI all the while it gets more threadbare? I yearn for the equivalent of the child's transitional object to help bridge the gap between practicing doctor and retired doctor identity. Had I been trained in the current era of molecular medicine, instead of the Freudian era, would I be fixating on the nature of my identity? At this stage of life, it would be considered sheer anachronistic folly. But I seem hell-bent on getting a tighter grip on who I am and what I am as my clock winds down—however anticlimactic that quest may be.

As I ruminate on my still indeterminate state, I am struck by the central-ity that tending to patients' identities played in my life and how that con-centration eclipsed any need to scrutinize my own. V. S. Pritchett, a literary giant of our time, finding himself in a somewhat analogous situation, has said that the way he was able to hold on to his identity as he aged was to write all the time, so as not to miss any part of himself and thereby avoid any semblance of occupational self-pity. Had I adopted Pritchett's credo along with that of another literary great, William Faulkner, who has said that in old age one must keep on keeping on (writing)—if I had continued to practice to the bitter end, mightn't I have avoided this preoccupation of pinning down my octogenarian identity? There is, of course, no answer, and in the end, everything gets unstitched anyway.

Remembering Jinx

Charles Helms, MD, PhD

The family's concern masked the beauty of that spring morning in the late 1940s. The boy had been ill about five days with a fever, chills, coryza, and myalgias. His temperature had reached 104° the previous night when his father had noticed the red, bumpy rash. The boy felt terrible. He was lethargic, unable to concentrate, lie still, or sleep. His appetite was off and his thirst prodigious, despite the large volumes of water, juice, and milk he consumed.

The boy's mother removed the thermometer from his mouth and, holding it at arm's length by the light of his bedroom window, she noted the temperature was 103.5°. "Still got the fever, Charlie," she reported. "Mind if we call Jinx?" The boy shrugged passively. She returned to the bed, hugged him close, kissed his forehead, and went to confer with her husband. The telephone call to John K, MD, or Jinx as his patients knew him, was made shortly afterward. He would drop by in the afternoon. The boy spent the rest of the morning dozing between doses of aspirin and glasses of juice.

Dr K was a short, stocky, muscular man with olive skin. He was an Armenian American, a second-generation member of a large contingent of Armenians who had immigrated to Watertown in the first half of the 20th century and who had succeeded in becoming part of the backbone of that Boston suburb through ambition and hard work. His lively dark brown eyes sparkled and jumped as he spoke, challenging you and holding your attention. His nose was prominent and hooked. He had short-cropped salt-and-pepper hair around the sides and back of his head. In contrast, the crown of this head was bare except for a layer of thin, gray fuzz. The scalp beneath was so shiny you could almost see your reflection in it. He was positively hirsute elsewhere, with thick eyebrows, tufts of hair protruding from his nose and ear canals, and a dense hair jacket from the base of his neck to his arms and small, sure hands.

Dr K's language was earthy, and his cursing was legendary. Even long-time patients would start or cringe at his epithets, but sooner or later, as the assault continued, they couldn't help but laugh, if only to relieve the tension. "Goddam!" "What the hell!" "Jesus Christ!" and "Son of a bitch!" peppered his conversation. Incredibly, Dr K was able to communicate empathy through such cursing! Equally incredible, patients seemed to understand and accept this unusual and idiosyncratic manner of registering their physical and emotional discomfort. Clearly, someone besides them was upset about their being ill, really upset! And that person could get away with language they could not. Thus, a typical Jinxian exchange might be:

Patient: Jinx, my sinuses are killing me! I feel lousy. I'm all worn out. I can't sleep and I can't do my housework.

Dr K: Well, Jesus Christ, Alice! You sound goddam uncomfortable!

Patient [stunned silence, slight wince]: Well, now that you put it that way, I guess I am. I mean, I guess I do.

Dr K: Damn right you do! You can't be any good to anyone, let alone yourself, feeling that way, Alice. Let's see if I can help. Anything else going on? Fever? Chills? Cold? Why aren't you sleeping?

So Jinx put on no airs and suffered none either. He clearly was not a doctor for the faint of heart, delicate of virtue, pompous, pious, or humorless, as all of these were usually left reeling by the barrage of gratuitous cursing. He was a blue-collar doc, a presence with an attitude.

This spring day Dr K's visit was typical Jinx. From the moment he entered the boy's room, he filled it with his characteristically noisy, energetic, and business-like movement, which stood in stark contrast to the family's quiet tip-toeing and suppressed worry. The room air positively swirled as he took off his sport coat, threw it on the boy's bed, raised the window shades, asked where "the hell" he could wash his hands, and then did so. An atmosphere of expectation built. Something was going to happen! As he wiped his hands with a bathroom towel, Jinx made small talk with the boy's parents.

Then he turned his attention to the boy, tossed the towel on the boy's bed over his coat, put his hands on his hips, and smiled warmly. "Hey, Charlie, my boy!" he exclaimed. "Where'd you get that goddam rash?" And a personal, one-on-one meeting was called to order in the midst of the group of four. Jinx sat down beside him quietly, listening carefully, and nodding encouragingly. As the boy spoke, Jinx examined him thoroughly from top to bottom. He interrupted the boy's rambling discourse and his own physical examination only for an occasional clarifying question ("Does the rash itch?"), an empathetic comment ("Damn, I'll bet that throat hurts!"), or a knowing affirmative grunt or nod ("Uh-huh! Yeah!"). At the conclusion of the boy's story and his examination, Jinx winked and said, "I want you to hear this." Then he placed the bell of his stethoscope over the boy's left breast, gave him the earpieces, and let him listen to the beating of his heart. "Sounds good, doesn't it?" Jinx said, nodding. The boy listened, too confused and awed by the lub-dubbing to answer. Speechless, he returned a nod and the instrument to Dr K with his first real smile in several days.

And then came the visit's finale. Jinx rummaged loudly through his instrument bag. Interrupting his search, he struck a serious but friendly pose and addressed the boy and his parents. "It's the goddam measles! Running like hell through the area and knocking the kids down. Charlie'll be sick for a few more days and then as right as rain. Give him plenty of fluids and whatever he'll eat." He resumed rummaging until he found what he was looking for and looked up with satisfaction. "A shot of penicillin will help him," he announced. A glass syringe emerged from a container in his bag. With a flourish he fit a needle to it and rummaged again to produce a vial of penicillin, the top of which he decapitated neatly with his thumb and forefinger in a fraction of a second. Then he introduced the needle into the vial and filled the syringe barrel noisily with fluid and bubbles. Dramatically he tossed the empty vial on the bed and forcefully expressed the bubbles and a little liquid in a fine jet across the room. It was a captivating and breathtaking performance.

Jinx paused, smiled, and held the syringe up to the light, admiring it, as one might a beautiful and expensive jewel. As if taking his cue, the boy lay down, turned his back to Dr K, and prepared for the inevitable. On his side with his knees flexed, he squeezed his eyes shut and held his breath. Then Jinx discretely and gently bared the boy's buttock, rubbed it vigorously with an alcohol-soaked cotton ball, and delivered the shot. With that, the boy relaxed, took a deep breath of alcohol vapor, and sat up again despite the evolving ache. Jinx scruffed the boy's hair, sat down beside him on the bed, and put his arm around his patient. He looked the boy in the eye. "You feel like crap now, Charlie," he said with restraint, for he would have used "shit" with an adult. "But, goddam it, you'll be better before you know it!" He then stood, patted the boy's back, packed his bag, put on his coat, and squeezed the mother's hand with a smile and emphasis. "Don't worry, Alice," he advised. He put his arm around the boy's father, a long-time friend, and exited the room. With Dr K's departure, the air in the room stopped swirling and the boy relaxed. He rubbed his throbbing buttock, a painful but real reminder that he'd begun to recover.

The boy in the story ultimately became an internist and teacher. He still reflects on the childhood event and the powerful impression that Jinx and his penicillin placebo made on his life. Clearly Dr K's use of penicillin to treat measles was unscientific and inappropriate, even for the late 1940s. Indeed, nowadays, the public is paying the price for inappropriate and appropriate antibiotic use over the years as antibiotic-resistant bacteria emerge and confound therapy.

Nevertheless, on that spring day, in that more innocent age nearly 50 years ago, Jinx had served the boy and his family well. His weaknesses in the science of medicine were fully matched by his strengths in its art.

Light in the Afternoon

J. Dennis Mull, MD, MPH

There was a remarkable stillness in the mosque. It did not seem possible that more than 200 people were there, seated on the floor in orderly rows, each waiting patiently for his or her special moment with the healer. A woman who looked as if she had been crying shuffled slowly forward. As she confided her story, the white-robed man with the piercing gaze leaned toward her, listening intently, and then touched her head, actually grasping it with one hand while he gently brushed her face with a peacock feather. He addressed a few words to her—words that I could not hear; he blew toward her three times; he handed her some herbs folded in a square of paper. Apparently this marked the end of the encounter, for she stood up, whispering her thanks, and another woman took her place.

Again the healer leaned forward and focused intently on his petitioner as she told her tale of fatigue and despair. Her young children had died one after the other before the age of 5, and her only grown son had not returned from a long absence; no one had enough to eat in her house. Although he must have heard such things a thousand times before, the healer seemed energized by her suffering. Putting his hands on her shoulders, he urged her not to give up hope. She was a special person, he said, and patience with her lot today would result in rewards tomorrow. "Wear this," he added with great conviction as he handed her a talisman with holy words written on it, "and you will feel better." The woman bowed her head in mute gratitude, and as she rose to leave, I noticed that she straightened her back with new resolve.

A shaft of white light broke through the ceiling, and the call of a mynah bird now interrupted the afternoon stillness. The crowd stirred slightly as the next patient, a man, leaned forward to confide his story, apparently not wanting anyone else to hear. The healer nodded and turned to the row of attentive, serious-faced assistants seated on the floor behind him. They handed him a cloth pouch. Taking from it, wrapped in a brown leaf, a remedy thought to restore sexual potency, he passed it on to his patient along with a few whispered remarks and a reassuring pat on the shoulder.

Then came a woman complaining of headaches. Her husband had taken a younger wife, she said, and had moved her toward the back of the house; she wanted a love charm to restore his interest. The healer spent a long time talking with this woman, probably 10 to 15 minutes, reassuring her that she had an important role in the family and that her advice was still needed. She had a right to receive equal treatment with the second wife, he advised, adding that he would talk with her husband about it if necessary. Meanwhile, at bedtime her husband should rub the back of her neck with a certain powder and the headaches would go away. By now glowing, the woman radiated a sense of relief and was gone.

And so it was, petitioner after petitioner came with their stories, revealing the most intimate secrets of their hearts to a man who listened attentively and seemed to care. I knew that outside the coolness of the mosque, theirs was a hot, dusty world essentially without hope, a world where almost no one could read or write, a monotonous world of hunger and hardship. How long would the momentary surge of well-being they had received from the healer last? I wondered. But then I recalled that it really didn't matter, for they could come back again whenever they wished.

The end of the session came in the late afternoon, with the ancient, melancholy call to 6-o'clock prayers reverberating as shadows fell. The patients who had not been seen were told that they could be first in line when the healer returned the next afternoon, and those who remained filed slowly out through the arched doorway. Later, after prayers, I drank tea with this quietly powerful man and asked about his past. He responded that some years before, he couldn't remember exactly when, he had started helping the great leader of the mosque. When the leader died, he hadn't tried to replace him spiritually, for that was done by someone else, but he had continued to offer medical care to those who sought it. In the morning, though, he was a simple baker who made bread and cookies for a living, some of which we were enjoying with our tea.

I reflected a bit on this, and on all that I had witnessed during the long afternoon. Noting the lateness of the hour, I asked him why he continued his work of healing, especially since he got nothing for it—why he took on such an enormous workload day after day. "Why? Because they need me," he answered. "Baking sometimes makes me tired, but healing never does. Baking, you see, is only what I *do*, while this is what I *am*."

So there it was: the healer was being healed, and in helping others to find hope, he was finding himself. With no medicines that modern science would consider effective, with no power but that of suggestion, touch, and a shared religious faith, he had succeeded in creating what Westerners would call an "ideal" therapeutic relationship, and, even more important, he was benefiting from it as much as his patients were.

As I left the mosque, constellations of stars were becoming visible in the summer sky, and in them I seemed to see the healer and his patients gleaming together through the darkness, each dependent on the other's feelings . . . each, like partners in a good love relationship, finding inspiration and mean ing in the chemistry of the transaction.

Today, at certain fortunate moments, I seem to see them still.

All in the Family

F amily plays an important role in the lives of physicians. Many have followed in the footsteps of a physician parent or relative—or have been influenced by a friend or mentor who is a physician—to become physicians themselves. Often these respected individuals simply lay the foundation for the demeanor of future physicians. In "A Doctor in Her House," a young physician learns—from observing an older and admired community doctor—that it is sometimes as important to know and understand the emotional and psychological (and even social) mien of her patients as it is to address their physical concerns. Or sometimes the testimonials of patients forge the steel of future generations of physicians, as in "Jerico Springs, Missouri" and "Ashes, Ashes." Perhaps the most difficult part of being a physician is treating (or not treating) one's family. This is dramatically realized in "A Conversation With My Mother," in which the author's mother asks him to help her end her life. Or the agony of knowing too much about your own child's precarious condition ("Message From Mahler," "For Everything a Blessing"). Whatever the relationship, "family" is for physicians multidimensional and unique.

R.K.Y.

Father's Day

Elaine Herrmann, RN, MPH

My father died of lung cancer in 1975. He was a physician.

Much has been written about the marriages of physicians—the satisfactions, the discord, the dynamics of these marriages. What of the effect of the physician's life on his or her children? What will they remember of their physician/father? What legacy does his quality of life leave them?

I doubt my father would ever have guessed my answer; less would he imagine the profound effect his life has had on mine. The wife chooses her husband; the child knows no choice. One's father is the norm against whom all other fathers are measured. Other children's fathers played ball with them, took them camping and on vacations. They taught their children fair play, an appreciation of nature, and the importance of family. Paradoxically, it was my father's absences that taught me something more, a stratum above: the meaning of responsibility, a commitment to purpose, and the necessity in the adult world to reconcile oneself with grace early on to the inevitable tragic injustices of life. A bitter lesson for a child? No, just a lesson. I knew no alternative. Furthermore, as poignant as was my father's occasional silent sorrow, so was his less frequent exhibition of joy.

What image first comes to mind at the recollection of my father? It is his dry, gnarled, loose-skinned hands, thumbnails deformed from childhood nail-biting. His primary tools for the practice of medicine were these square hands with distended veins that palpated abdomens, axillae, and necks. They sutured lacerations, bandaged wounds, and delivered narcotic relief from the pain that usurps personality, restoring dignity to his patient. They removed splinters from elderly skin and soothed the small child's burns. His competent hands inserted IV catheters and intubated airways with refined precision, but they also mixed compost with the soil of the brilliant begonias he loved. They built our doll beds. He spoke little; his hands spoke for him and about him.

Often I accompanied him on Saturday afternoons on his house calls and hospital rounds. After rescuing me from my piano lessons, he called on patients while I waited in the car, where I pored over his journals. The graphic photos of trauma and skin eruptions fascinated me. I doubt he ever knew how much I looked forward to looking at the journals. He was less likely to question my interest than he was concerned that I not crumple the x-rays in their pumpkin-yellow Kodak covers or overturn Mrs Jones' urine specimen in the bag on the floor that was destined for the hospital lab. Waiting for him in the hospital lobby, I spent hours reading worn magazines and playing hopscotch on the black and white linoleum-square floor. I felt my patience rewarded when he would lead me into the inner sanctum of Radiology's darkroom, at the center of a blackened, inwardly spiraling narrow hallway, to show me developing x-ray films.

More often than not, the telephone dictated that he leave in the middle of the night to make a house call or to go to the hospital. After wakening to the ringing phone, I would listen to hear the front door close in the dark. Lying alert in bed, I watched the headlight beams sweep across my windowshade as the car backed down the driveway. I would then sleep fitfully, waiting to see the lights cross in the other direction, indicating he was safely home.

In the summer, patients sometimes paid him in fruit, boxes of which he would bring home to can, always a monumental undertaking. He transformed our kitchen into a rudimentary central supply station, with jars and lids cleaned and boiling on the stove, pits and skins tidily disposed of, the whole room dense with steam. Fearing disruption of his system, he let no one help him. Throughout the year, he exchanged jars of the end product with patients who also canned, and critiques of each others' preserves were solicited. Occasionally a truck would pull up to the side of the house and firewood would be unloaded and stacked, another form of payment for services rendered.

Surely such methods of payment would have frequently introduced the subject of money and income. On the contrary, finances were rarely discussed. Leery of the concept of money making money through investments and disdainful of business, he passed on to his children a boredom with business as a career.

At the dinner table we rarely spoke of politics or current events. Instead, my father asked about our classes, and not infrequently we were involuntary students of lectures on such topics as anatomy. Using a roasted leg of lamb or a baked chicken, he demonstrated ball-and-socket, hinged, and gliding joints. Pork chops were served with metal utensils that I learned as a teenager were delivery forceps. Aside from his extensive reading of medical journals, European history, and English literature (the result of the curse—or blessing—of insomnia), his only hobby was gardening. Each morning for 25 years my mother cut roses for my father to take to elderly patients in the hospital and to nurses' stations. To this day, there are plants and shrubs discreetly tied to stakes with his clear plastic tubing.

Before the availability of emergency rooms such as they are today, patients, particularly children, would be brought to our house in the evening or on weekends, where they would be examined under good light, with my nurse/mother's assistance, on white sheets spread on the dining room table. Coming into the house from climbing trees, we were promptly ushered down the hall to our rooms to give the patient's family privacy.

Even as a young child I had the greatest regard for what my father was. Completely unaware at such an age of the social ramifications of being a physician's child, I was simply grateful, though I could not have articulated it, that my father did not have a routine 8 to 5 job, after which he came home, watched the news, drank a beer, and washed the car. My father did not have a job; he had a purposefully dedicated life.

In November 1974, my father treated several patients for a viral gastritis. He'd also contracted it, he thought. The patients improved. He worsened. Diagnosed with metastatic disease of the liver, he practiced medicine while undergoing chemotherapy until he was too weak to continue. He entered the hospital the day after he closed his practice. My searing grief upon removing his name sign from the front of his office is vivid yet. This one cruel task most signified the imminence of his death. After a brief remission, he deteriorated rapidly the week after Easter. My mother, my sister, and I cared for him at home, watching hour by hour the disfiguring deterioration, until, face and abdomen swollen, he hovered on the edge of consciousness. What little he muttered in his metastatic confusion reflected a lifetime of medical practice: "Did she have the flat plate? . . . Did the lab call back with his results?" With time running out, I was desperate to tell him what he meant to me. As I started to speak, leaning intently from my chair toward his pillow, he opened his eyes and weakly announced, "I'm not dying today." End of that conversation. Within two days he was comatose. Finally, at 5 o'clock on an April afternoon, over the granite hands that buttressed his jaw cascaded a brief maroon rivulet from between his gray lips, heralding the end of the wellspring of my inspiration: this man, this physician, my father.

Albert J. Herrmann, MD
1906-1975

Ashes, Ashes

L. Stewart Massad, MD

It is only 4 o'clock, but this late in November the dark comes early. The sky is overcast, and from the fields the west wind carries the smell of rain into my old hometown. This morning I picked up my wife and sons at the little airport there. Now we stand about the funeral parlor in our best black, alone with our thoughts, waiting for calling hours to begin.

In death my father is unrecognizable. His hands—physician's hands, once so busy—are folded on his chest inside the open casket. His sardonic smile is gone, and the mortician has painted over any trace of former joy, grief, anger, or concern. I cannot bear to look at him.

On the way from the airport, we stopped by his house, the house where he and then I grew up. Nothing is left but a black cellar hole full of twisted cable, broken pipe, shattered tile, a sink, burned framing. The apple tree that we planted in the front yard 43 years ago is dead too, withered by the blaze. The autumn lawn, black and gray with ash, still wears the muddy scars of firefighters' boots, truck tires, hoses, and the wheels of the gurney.

The first firefighters on the scene found him, before flames took over the old Queen Anne. My father died on the stairwell, killed not by the flames but by the smoke. Except for college, medical school, and the war, he had lived all his life in that house. He was a small-town doctor, a general practitioner with an office beside the hospital four blocks away. Time was when he saw 30 people there each day, rounded on an inpatient or two or three, and stopped to visit the homebound before winding his own way home. His style was something out of the past. He never bought a computer, wrote out notes and orders longhand, employed a single secretary; my mother was his nurse. Content to diagnose with his hands, his stethoscope, a blood pressure cuff, and a microscope, he had no time for acronyms, scans, or profiles. He guarded his practice, nurtured it, treasured it. But the past is past, and six years ago he retired, forced to give up his practice by things he never understood: paperwork, technology, specialists, my mother's death.

I have been in town two days. Yesterday I met with my father's lawyer, his accountant, the coroner, the funeral home director. There has been little for me to do: although I am pushing 50, they all are of my father's generation, knew me as a boy, have everything arranged.

When I was a child, it was assumed that I would take over my father's practice, as he had my grandfather's. But I carry too many memories of what my father's practice cost: his chair at dinner empty, late-night calls that drove him out in bitter weather, long walks home from lost ball games he never managed to attend, my mother's loneliness and my own. Then, too, I knew my old man. I knew his way was passing and didn't want to fight to change him, knowing we'd both lose. And I knew how he loved treating this town's tangled troubles. I have always been different.

When the doors of the funeral home open, I am at the end of the receiving line. My aunt and her husband arrive: we share condolences, kisses on the cheek. Old men who in the morning will be pallbearers put out their cigarettes and come in from the hall. A humped old woman in a red wool coat hobbles up, squeezes my hand, and confides, "Back in high school, your father was the cutest." More old people pass, telling me I look just like the old man—or just like my mother. I thank them for their sympathy and watch as they step to the casket to stand a moment, a moment more, and then move on.

A crowd forms in the hall. The funeral home director, impressed, crosses the room to speak to me about the line that winds out the door and round the block. Who are all these people? I recognize a few: the captain of my high school football team, now heavy and gray, my father's secretary. Many were my father's friends. All, it seems, were his patients.

Women introduce sheepish teenagers my father delivered. I hear about the hazards of farming: cuts and bruises, sprains and fractures my father fixed. A man my age tells me of the tumor my father found, a bowel cancer caught in time. The line waits while his story goes on and on, until he breaks down in tears and it is I who am consoling him. Then it seems half the room is teary: the young insurance agent whose diabetes my father diagnosed, the mother whose child survived epiglottitis, the bank teller with arthritis, the daughter of an Alzheimer's patient. I meet the car mechanic with bad coronaries, shake the hands of American Legionnaires with lung disease, a tailor with gout, and the pharmacist who, like my mother once, is beautiful and has lupus. I look into the eyes of those whose tales, though untellable, I know from things my father told me: the cirrhotic painter pregnant with ascites, the waitress with slash marks beneath her watchband.

The procession goes on and on. My wrist grows sore. My hand grows tired. Till well past 7 I am the focus of the whole town's grief. I catch in their voices a hint of their reproach—or perhaps only my own guilt—that I did not take my father's place, that they have been left to doctors who are well intentioned and competent but not their own.

I thought I understood my home, but I see now that I never did, never really tried, was too eager to get away. Then I realize that I never really understood my father either, or why he loved the work that punished him. The answer is in the faces of his patients tonight.

Still, it is too late for regrets. My father is dead, his home is ash, and medicine has changed forever. In the morning will be the funeral. I will say his eulogy, though his truest tribute was tonight. My father will be buried, and yet as long as the people I met tonight survive, he will remain part of this town.

When the line winds to its end, when the mortician locks the door, I stand on the concrete walk in the splash of porch light under the vast black prairie sky, alone.

Haying

Harriet A. Squier, MD, MA

When it is sunny in June, my father gets in his first cutting of hay. He starts on the creek meadows, which are flat, sandy, and hot. They are his driest land. This year, vacationing from my medical practice, I returned to Vermont to help him with the haying.

The heft of a bale through my leather gloves is familiar: the tautness of the twine, the heave of the bale, the sweat rivers that run through the hay chaff on my arms. This work has the smell of sweet grass and breeze. I walk behind the chug and clack of the baler, moving the bales into piles so my brother can do the real work of picking them up later. As hot as the air is, my face is hotter. I am surprised at how soon I get tired. I take a break and sit in the shade, watching my father bale, trying not to think about how old he is, how the heat affects his heart, what might happen.

This is not my usual work, of course. My usual work is to sit with patients and listen to them. Occasionally I touch them, and am glad that my hands are soft. I don't think my patients would like farmer calluses and dirty hands on their tender spots. Reluctantly I feel for lumps in breasts and testicles, hidden swellings of organs and joints, and probe all the painful places in my patients' lives. There are many. Perhaps I am too soft, could stand calluses of a different sort.

I feel heavy after a day's work, as if all my patients were inside me, letting me carry them. I don't mean to. But where do I put their stories? The childhood beatings, ulcers from stress, incapacitating depression, fears, illness? These are not my experiences, yet I feel them and carry them with me. I search out these stories in my patients, try to reorganize them, try to find healthier meanings. I spent the week before vacation crying.

The hay field is getting organized. Piles of three and four bales are scattered around the field. They will be easy to pick up. Dad climbs, tired and lame, from the tractor. I hand him a jar of ice water, and he looks with satisfaction on his job just done. I'll stack a few more bales and maybe drive the truck for my brother. My father will have some appreciative customers this winter, as he sells his bales of hay.

I've needed to feel this heaviness in my muscles, the heat on my face. I am taunted by the simplicity of this work, the purpose and results, the definite boundaries of the fields, the dimensions of the bales, for illness is not defined by the boundaries of bodies; it spills into families, homes, schools, and my office, like hay tumbling over the edge of the cutter bar. I feel the rough stubble left in its wake. I need to remember the stories I've helped reshape, new meanings stacked against the despair of pain. I need to remember the smell of hay in June.

Last Rounds

Joseph T. Martorano, MD

I cradle my father carefully in my arms. His chin rests against my right shoulder as the physician slips the long thoracentesis needle into his back, searching for the cause of his inability to swallow food.

The physician's eyes evade mine. We are both 50 years old and between us have practiced medicine for a collective half-century. My father is a 78-year-old general practitioner. Half a century earlier he caught his father's leg during an amputation for diabetes. Together the three of us complete a century of medicine.

Finally the bitter answer comes. Ironically, my father, who has spent a lifetime railing against cigarette smoking, is to die of a rare lung cancer. We settle down. Even as we tell him the brutal diagnosis, I learn that a doctor dies differently.

My father's initial response is muted anguish, but quickly his professional pride takes over. "I knew I was right." Months before complicated technology finally located the lesion, he had turned his own formidable diagnostic skills inward and informed us he had cancer. We had tried to prove him wrong.

There is little time for self-pity. He has spent 50 caring years alleviating the pain of others. He isn't about to stop now. His final task is to lessen our pain.

Never once does he mention that as a GP he was long ago forced from hospital practice by a bureaucracy favoring specialization. Nor does he mention that the world has become an increasingly hostile place for the aging solo practitioner. Instead he remains an observer, astutely monitoring his own case. He is a far wiser and more learned physician than most. Fifty long years without backup have made him totally independent, with an incredible storehouse of medical knowledge. He continues to want to take care of himself, but it is not easy. The daily choices are harder. There is confusion as to when to be a doctor and when to be a patient. My father has lived a frugal but generous life. It becomes increasingly harder for him to justify the countless expensive procedures and elaborate nursing charges to prolong the myth of possibility. Wisely he chooses chemotherapy and radiation, more for the hope they give us than for himself.

In a life totally devoted to medicine, the endless demands of his practice left little time for family, and we were almost strangers until I graduated from medical school. At that point our relationship developed, and we became the closest of friends. Eventually I too moved out from the hospital and chose to practice alone. He is the one physician I talk to every day. I frequently ask his advice. But we disagree on what medicine has become and how we should relate to it.

My father embraced medicine with an almost religious fervor while I work in a more business-oriented way, experiencing anger and frustration with increasing government regulations and demanding third-party compliance. I am ten years removed from daily hospital work. But now, as a daily visitor, I become an observer watching with microscopic scrutiny. The technological changes are incredible. Everything is computerized electronics and sophisticated radiographic techniques. Yet, paradoxically, the changes only make the days more agonizing, filling them with hundreds of complex, often bitter decisions on just how much technology can be used to defer death. My father has attended thousands of deaths, experiences that sharpen his sense of inevitability and give him a different sensibility that visibly increases the already intense bonding with the young house staff. The doctors reach out during rounds and gently touch his body. Surprisingly, my father accepts their compassion gratefully. I have forgotten how concerned physicians can be, compared with my highly successful, but emotionally clumsy, business friends.

As time passes, I notice that many of the medical staff are overly interested in my two sons, his grandchildren. At first I mistake it as compassion; but then I recognize it as something else, a question about the future. Medicine is perceived as dying. Will my sons, with a medical background spanning close to a century, choose the profession, or is there a better present choice?

As his condition weakens, in a single day my father, who for most of his life charged five dollars for a house call, unknowingly spends hundreds of dollars on useless technology to help him die. My father and his kind of medicine are both dying. There will be no more house calls, no more goods offered in lieu of money for payment. Instead there will be only an avalanche of paperwork, malpractice worries, and fear. The cancer killing our profession is as malignant as the dread oat cells eroding my father's body.

The Japanese say you only die once: therefore, you must practice every day to get it right. Somehow the practice of medicine has always been entwined with the practice of dying. My father does it well, suffering without complaint, grateful for the smallest amelioration of his discomfort.

Rounds continue on, now passing us by. There is little to be said, there are few tears left to spend. When my father can no longer swallow, we must pay attention to the newspapers. Each visitor takes on heraldic importance; after a while each becomes family. Each relationship has to be special, each moment becomes something of value. But there is not enough time.

The radiation unexpectedly shrinks the tumor. My father gratefully swallows small pieces of soft cheese, the first food he has tasted in months. The next day he throws up continuously, in excruciating pain. His eyes seek mine; the doctor has reached his final clinical decision. My father says, "I can't take any more. It is time to go," and he steps into the shadow to where he caught his father's leg half a century earlier. He dies peacefully with me alone at his bedside.

At the grave site, as I embrace my two sons, memories of the tearful concern in the eyes of my colleagues flood back. The message clears.

Medicine is still very much alive, but it lives not so much in the frontiers of the new technology, which too often only painfully prolongs the entrance of death, as in the hearts of the physicians. We will persist because of the deep compassion we develop in caring for life while living with death. My inheritance is a rich one: the privilege of being able to care for others. It is this pride that transcends death that my father and I share best.

It is the purest of loves.

. . . For My Father

Khalid J. Awan, MD, FPAMS

A physician is, or at least is supposed to be, fully versed in handling the professional, social, and even spiritual aspects of death. But the sudden death of my father last year made bare the facets of this phenomenon to which I was oblivious before. I was overwhelmed by apprehensions, regrets, and grief that no professional expertise could eradicate or ease. My father's presence, his advice, his prayers were an invincible shield between me and all adversity, and because of it I fearlessly took on every challenge that came my way. After his death, there quietly appeared a strange reluctance, a caution in my approach. In Whittemore's words, "With his passing I was abruptly stripped of any illusions of my own immortality; no longer might I comfort myself with the thought that he was next in line ahead of me. For any boy, that is one of his father's silent functions—to stand as a shield between his son and the abyss."

My first impression of my father is that of a stranger in uniform standing in our doorway. It was the time of World War II, and he had volunteered to serve. Soon after the war, he agreed to lead an expedition to take over a military post for our country in the snowy mountains of Kashgar. By the time he came home, I was already 5. Our relationship began with my having this odd feeling of strangeness about him, but his noninsistent and gentle approach gradually reassured me. What really made me comfortable was my child's eye keenly noticing how those who met my father even in the street greeted him with respect and a smile.

Nor was discipline lacking in his parenting. I was a handful in my teens, and had it not been for proper disciplining, I surely would have neglected my studies. A mulberry tree stood next to our house, and occasionally my father had to resort to the use of one of its branches to set me right. After my graduation from medical school, whenever I and my father walked by that tree, we would look at each other and burst out laughing. My childhood friends still joke that were it not for that mulberry tree, I wouldn't be a doctor today.

My father also was the role model in my professional conduct. His utter lack of greed and his intense concern for his patients nurtured in me the desire to become a scrupulous physician. He was fiercely self-dependent and would rather limit his needs than be under obligation to others. This taught me the true meaning and value of self-respect. For years, when I still was a boy in school, it was my father's routine to play chess each evening with the Nawab of Kalabagh (in Pakistan). When later the Nawab became the governor of our state, I, at the prodding of my friends, thoughtlessly asked my father if he would get me an appropriate medical posting from the governor. "No, Son," he made it emphatically clear, "if I do this, all my friends will think I foster relationships for personal gain. The quickest way to lose respect in the eyes of others is to bring them your needs." I can still hear him saying, "Faith in God and self-reliance mean that the need you cannot meet yourself isn't your need."

Yet, when it came to others, I don't remember him ever saying no to anyone who sought his help. I so many times saw him knocking on the office door of even the lowliest of bureaucrats to plead for a job for some poor family man. Many of his patients were country people who traveled miles to seek his help. He gave them free medicines, and when any of them needed longer care, he put them up in a spare room attached to our home. In those days there weren't many hospitals. My mother looked after their meals and other needs, and when they were ready to go home, my father bought their train or bus tickets. This happened so often that for a long time I thought it was a required part of medical practice. His death took away from the people around him an ever-willing benefactor; from me, my earthly wellspring of guidance and steadfastness.

Despite his weaknesses—he was a pitiful money manager and a chain smoker 'til his last day—I gradually came to believe that if he set his heart to it, there wasn't a thing in the world he couldn't take care of. This belief in the goodness and greatness of this man whom everyone admired had coated my subconscious with an impervious layer of security, which his death suddenly peeled away. Even throughout my adult life, I felt greatly reassured after consulting my father. My confidence in his wisdom, experience, and sincerity was so deep-seated that I never felt even the slightest embarrassment when he drew my attention to some silly flaw in my reasoning or approach to a problem.

My apprehensions upon his loss arose from my losing his guidance that in my mind never missed its mark, my regrets from not having been there with him all that time, my grief from losing someone who loved me so dearly yet so selflessly. The thought of to whom I would now open myself when plagued by fears and doubts relentlessly gnawed on my mind. Because my father's wisdom and experience are there no more to boost me, a more deliberate behavior has quietly displaced the impetuosity in me. A keener awareness of my own mortality brought on by his passing has erased from my mind every temptation to place any expedient consideration before honesty or self-esteem. Becoming reft of his support has induced me to rely subconsciously on what he imparted to my character.

As the shock of my father's death began to wear off, my attention became more focused on my own role as the leading link in the life chain of my family. I now realize more acutely that the good that my father had must now live through me. I came to see that for a son, the son-father relationship is an honorable debt that when paid honestly perpetuates happiness. The question of how one pays a dead father the debt one owes has brought to my view the flip side of life's coin, revealing that one pays to one's children the debt one owes to one's father. That is how good is passed on from one generation to the next. I found in me an unconstrained willingness to be more attentive to the needs of my children, more eager to extend to them my hand in help, and more tolerant of their youthful antics.

I am also almost imperceptibly acquiring a demeanor with my patients that was so characteristic of my father. Where I used to feel strain on hearing the clinically unnecessary and repetitious details some patients have the habit of giving, I now find myself much more willing to listen. I have become more forebearing with the excuses my patients bring me, and like my father, I also try to extend nonprofessional assistance to those who need it. But such good has its own reward. No amount of money and no amount of hard work can bring the kind of happiness I felt when I drove home an elderly patient whose ride had left him stranded in my office. Even in his death, my father has taught me how to be a better father and a better man. An intelligent person would learn from anyone's death.

To ponder the philosophical and spiritual perceptions of death is an efficient balm to the bereaved's grief and depression. This is not necessarily restricted to one's religious beliefs, for a rational analysis of day-to-day observations on life and death may also bring solace by imparting a clearer understanding of this reality. Death is not the end. Socrates, though not very vocal about God, was totally convinced of the immortality of the soul. Hence, when authorities hand Socrates the cup of hemlock, Crito asks him in Plato's *Phaedo*, "How shall we bury you?" "However you please, if you can catch me, and I do not get away from you," replies Socrates with a gentle laugh. Clearly, he was speaking of one's true self, his soul, which on leaving the prison of flesh becomes free of all confines, and never perishes.

Death is a transformation. Faith is an indispensable source of comfort and courage when material means fail us. Day after day in our professional practice, we see the comfort that turning to faith brings to patients with diseases that have reached beyond our ability to treat. Both faith and reason helped me overcome my irreplaceable loss and made me a better human in the process.

Yes, my father is dead, but his existence has not ended. He continues to live, in Heaven in reality, and in our hearts symbolically. I am sad no more. My bosom is still full of his love, my deeds still add to his good name, and my prayers are still filled with supplications for his salvation. And I add to my every prayer, Bless too, O Almighty, all the caring fathers, those living with us on this earth and those living with God's promise in the hereafter.

Jerico Springs, Missouri

Brent Swager

I could've died. I guess you know that." The heavy-set woman had me cornered in the Dr Scholl's section of the Rexall and, having ascertained that I was indeed Doc Bannister's "boy," was doggedly reciting one of Grandpa's medical miracles. She struggled with her baggy sweatshirt until a jiggling, puckered underbelly flopped out. She dug through folds of flesh until she located a small, slick scar.

"Right 'air." She stretched the loose skin tight for better viewing. "Doc took it out, right on the . . ."

"Kitchen table," I finished. The memory had come rushing back to me so strongly that I could smell iodine and alcohol, mixed with the greasy odor of the Walshes' kitchen.

———

It was hot in the farmhouse. Heat crackled off the tin roof, causing me to start with every pop it made. Outside the sagging screen door, chickens squabbled over a hard-backed June bug. Mr Walsh paced the floor behind me and murmured to himself, hawked and swallowed nois-ily until Grandpa Doc noticed him and told him he could wait outside. Mrs Walsh, 20 years younger then, lay on the kitchen table, feverish and moaning.

I was only 8 years old, but after a summer spent as my grandfather's shadow, I felt it my rightful place to be involved and strengthened my case by always holding the cracked brown leather bag, whose contents I had memorized and could dole out with the same palm-slapping efficiency as a surgical nurse.

Just that morning, as Grandpa hummed and smoked his morning Roi-Tan while scrambling eggs, I had tonged the gleaming steel instruments out of the steamer and had named each one under his watchful eye as I laid them out on a sterile towel. Grandpa quizzed me as I worked.

"What do you recommend for an open wound?" Grandpa asked as he stirred diced bell peppers into the eggs.

"Antibiotics," I answered, dutiful as any third-year student.

"And whose motto is 'Standard of the World'?"

"Cadillac," I responded correctly. Grandpa liked to keep you on your toes.

When the telephone rang, Grandpa left me to stir the eggs while he talked.

"Get my bag," he whispered, covering the mouthpiece with one hand. He closed his eyes and nodded into the receiver, saying, "Yes. We'll be there in ten minutes, Mr Walsh."

I ran next door to the small, concrete-block clinic Grandpa kept, grabbed the doctor kit, raced back to the house, scooped towel, instruments, and two bottles of penicillin into the bag, and bolted out the kitchen door as Grandpa shut down the eggs and gargled Listerine in the bathroom. I fumbled with the keys but got the Cadillac started as Grandpa twanged out the screen door, disturbing Tom Dooley off a favorite porch rocker, and bounded down the front steps. Tom Dooley wagged his tail hopefully and followed. Grandpa opened the Cadillac's back door.

"Okay," he told the fat cocker spaniel, "you can come, but hurry up." Tom huffed in and sat panting and drooling in the back seat.

Gravel pinged off the Cadillac's undercarriage as we rocketed down back country roads toward the Walsh farm. Grandpa's usual hum had changed to hoot-toot and snatches of Elvis songs, indicating that this was something serious, so when the car slid to a stop, I was ready and, with the clanking doctor bag bouncing against my leg, beat fat old Tom Dooley to the front door, ducking through on Grandpa's heels. Tom nosed open the battered screen door and followed, flopping down under the kitchen table.

The light was better in the kitchen. Grandpa examined Mrs Walsh under the timid glare of the bedroom's single light bulb, which dangled from a frayed black cord in the middle of the ceiling, while Mr Walsh and I cleared the table. Grandpa bundled his patient in the bedsheets and carried her in. He rolled up his sleeves and stood over a tin pail that the Walshes used for a sink while I poured yellow iodine over his hands. He snapped on rubbery latex gloves and finally noticed Mr Walsh pacing and clearing his throat, in orbit behind us.

"You can wait outside, Mr Walsh," he said. "We'll be okay in here."

Mr Walsh bolted out the screen door in obvious relief, scattering the curious chickens across the dusty front yard. They regrouped immediately and gathered 'round the front to peer in again.

"Lidocaine?" Grandpa's low voice brought me back to the task at hand.

It wasn't my first syringe, but it was the first one under pressure. Mrs Walsh had been covered with bath towels and a sheet so that only a small portion of her was available to the eye and, finally, the knife. My hands shook as I nervously drew up the deadening drug and handed it to the doctor.

It was over so breathlessly fast that at first I wondered if I'd actually witnessed it. With my own two wide-open eyes, I'd looked inside another human being. The fouled appendix lay bloated and bloody streaked on a towel on the kitchen table. Grandpa hummed as he sewed up Mrs Walsh and thanked me for my assistance.

"Go tell Mr Walsh he can come on back," he smiled at me, and I sailed out the door, scattering the nosy chickens once more. I found Mr Walsh hunkered down on the shady side of the springhouse, whittling a hickory whistle with his buck knife. He handed it to me as I walked up—payment for my small part, I guess—and followed me back to the house.

As I gathered up the soiled instruments, Grandpa gave Mrs Walsh her penicillin shots, the most painful part of the whole experience from what I could tell, if noise was an indicator, and gave Mr Walsh strict instructions and a promise that he'd drive out tomorrow to check on things.

"You still keep chickens?" I asked now, and blushed, thinking I should have asked after Mr Walsh first. Mrs Walsh hugged me to her huge bosom and laughed.

"He was the best doctor ever," she wiped a jolly tear away. "Best ever," she repeated, and waddled away to fill her prescription, leaving me standing in the corn and bunion relief aisle with Grandpa's ghost chuckling beside me.

A Doctor in Her House

Bernadine Z. Paulshock, MD

He's 75 or 80 years old now and retired from private practice, although there are still lots of patients and physicians in our suburban community who remember Dr M well. When the local newspaper published an article about him recently, the reporter concentrated mostly on Dr M's experience as a young pediatrician in training. When he was an intern, polio epidemics were rampant, and the Boston hospitals were filled with "iron lungs." He remembers when Franklin Delano Roosevelt was stricken with polio. He attended the Rome conference where Jonas Salk and Albert Sabin first talked about their successful vaccine stories.

And one day, without especially trying to, the pediatrician Dr M made a true physician of me. It was a long time ago, only a few months after I began to practice internal medicine. One of my patients called and asked that I come see her. She was too ill to leave her house, she said—one of her kids was sick too. She thought it was chickenpox because her other two children had recently had it. I wasn't overjoyed at having to make a home visit, but she was a new patient (as were all my patients), and I hoped to please her, hoped even that she'd tell her friends about me.

She lived on a busy street where parking may not have been legal and would certainly have been dangerous. I remember that I parked my car in the supermarket lot that bordered her backyard and walked around to the front door, which was unlocked.

My patient was in bed upstairs. She looked ill, but her temperature was only 101° (those were Fahrenheit days). She had no vesicles or pustules on her oral mucous membranes, nor any signs of respiratory tract involvement. Her neck was supple. She certainly had chickenpox, but the lesions seemed limited to her skin.

Only one of her three little children was sick. Sucking his thumb, he huddled in an armchair in her room, clutching a very grungy small teddy bear and a torn blanket in one hand and scratching steadily with his other. His face was peppered with chickenpox and he was scratching them all. I asked about him, and she told me her pediatrician was coming later to check all three of the children. Dr M: I recognized his name and was impressed.

The other two kids were playing Pick Up Sticks at the foot of her bed. I had never thought of Pick Up Sticks as a violent game, but theirs was. I asked them to beat it to another room so I could listen to their mother's chest, which was clear, and to her heart. She had very mild tachycardia, regular rhythm, nothing of concern.

"Where is your husband?" I asked. "You really need him."

"Milwaukee. Company business. He won't be home for three more days."

Wilmington, Delaware, is a company town. Its laboratories are always being refilled with bright young scientists, often just out of graduate school. They come from all over the country. I had lived in Wilmington for a year or so before meeting anyone who had been born there. I knew better than to ask if my patient had a mother or sister to help her. Obviously she didn't, or they would have been there already.

"Does your husband know you're sick?" I asked.

"I told him," she replied. "He said he never knew adults could get childhood diseases like chickenpox. He said it must be because my mother and father sheltered me too carefully. I guess they did."

"Aspirin," I advised. (Yes, I did. It was routine then, and none of us knew any better.) "And lots of fluids like fruit juice. And extra rest." The kids were by now back at their ferocious game.

"They had it first," she said. "Tommy and I are the second wave. I do wish I had had chickenpox when I was a kid."

Kicking aside a toy that somehow had gotten wedged in the door, I let myself out, reclaimed my car, and drove off. I felt a bit uneasy because I realized that what she really needed was not a doctor but a husband or a mother. I knew I was going to feel guilty about billing her.

I was sufficiently concerned that I called the next day to ask how she was. I was going to suggest that a visiting nurse stop by to check on her.

"I'm a lot better today," she said. "I just gave the kids a real lunch . . . chicken sandwiches. Yesterday I let them eat cold cereal with marshmallow paste on it. And Tommy is some better too. Dr M gave him medicine for his itching, some samples he had in his bag, and Tommy's stopped scratching his pox and he also ate a chicken sandwich.

"And Dr M did something else for us," she marveled. "Something really great." I still ask myself, was her voice even the tiniest bit accusing? I don't think so.

"After he left here, Dr M walked over to the supermarket and brought back some groceries: milk, a quart of juice, a barbecued chicken, some bananas. I was so surprised! And he wouldn't even let me pay him. Wasn't that terrific of him? He really is one terrific doctor."

Why hadn't *I* thought of getting supper for her and her kids? The idea of making sure they had some supper should have occurred to me, a mother. But it hadn't. I had been preoccupied with trying to recall all I'd ever heard or read about chickenpox in adults. I knew the disease made adults sicker than children, but unless they got pneumonia or meningitis they usually got better without sequelae.

Dr M knew that too. In fact, he knew more about chickenpox than I'll ever know. But he also saw that the kids were hungry and their mother needed help. He fed them and helped her.

And I did not.

My patient's chickenpox cleared quickly and left her with no sequelae, but it did me. And I've been a better physician for it. Years later, I told Dr M about the episode. He didn't even remember it, but I do, and I always will.

Dr M began to refer me his "outgrown" patients. I was happy and proud to get his adolescents, except for the ones with first or middle names of John or Johanna, those who had been named after him. They seemed too uniquely heavy a responsibility and made me a little uncomfortable, for I already knew I couldn't measure up to Dr M.

Message From Mahler

Dan Gehlbach, MD

I can remember reading the essay on Gustav Mahler's *Ninth Symphony* by Lewis Thomas and feeling puzzled, as though I had missed something important. Written by a man who had just learned from his physician that he would soon succumb to a fatal heart ailment, the symphony has been viewed as Mahler's despairing swan song as he attempts to come to grips with a premature death. Thomas, however, could not listen to the symphony without envisioning the agony of a global holocaust, as though the individual chords represented waves of thermonuclear death raining from the skies. Try as I might, playing my tape over and over, I could not hear the blasts of the bombs or the death rattle of the world. Even with the volume full blast on my Walkman, surrounded by the swirling clash of the movement's most violent assault, I knew there would come the gentle and reassuring refrain from the strings, singing of peace, of hope, of rest. I could not hear death.

We were joking as we came out from the C-section, as we often did after the unspoken tension involved in bringing another life into the world. Stationed at the eastern border of West Germany, I was now on loan to this hospital on the other side of Germany, filling a temporary slot until the arrival of the next crop of physicians. Being away from my family for two weeks was never pleasant, but we had survived before. When serving the jealous "mistresses" of both medicine and the military, one had no choice.

My replacement for call caught me by the arm but held me with an uneasy stare as she motioned me into the chair. I knew that look; I had used it before (too many times) as I discussed with a patient a path report that wasn't benign, or said softly but professionally to a weeping couple there was nothing more I could do. But this time the look was for me.

"Your hospital just called. I'm afraid your son has had another asthma attack, a bad one. They say he's stable on the ventilator now, and they think the seizures will stop soon. . . . Your wife is pretty shook up."

The next 30 minutes remain a blur, although the necessary phone calls must have been made to release me from duty, to find me a quick way back. There was none. The chopper wasn't available, the duty truck wasn't leaving for several hours, I didn't have a car because I had come by train. It was a six-hour train ride, counting the two changes on the way. I asked the cab driver to hurry as we drove to the station.

This was vacation time in Germany, and the trains were packed with happy, sweating vacationers. There were no seats open on any of the trains, so I crouched in the corner with my duffel bag, at times pacing nervously in front of the window. My neighbors eyed me suspiciously as I alternated between spates of cursing and praying under my breath. My fists clenched involuntarily as I remembered the other family crises when I had been away or on call and unable to respond. Visions of my 7-year-old's happy-go-lucky grin were replaced by a pale face lost behind the maze of tubes and wires I was all too familiar with. The train couldn't go fast enough; I felt I was going insane.

We were more than halfway there when I put on my Walkman in a vain attempt at distraction. The familiar strains of Mahler's *Ninth* began to calm me as I tried to concentrate on the green countryside passing by and forget the cruel truth that awaited me. It was then that I first heard it. Entering the music almost silently, it provoked a slight disharmony that was at first barely discernible, but grew steadily stronger and more powerful. I sat transfixed as the tempo gradually lifted me into a swirling maelstrom of discord and destruction, of violence and despair. Here was the death that Mahler was forced to confront, the death witnessed so clearly by Thomas, the death I had pretended not to see. Nor was this the distant death I discussed so professionally with my patients, which I had viewed before from a sympathetic but detached physician's viewpoint. Instead it seemed as though I were face to face with a menacing figure whose shadowy features were distorted by a hatred and loathing that were directed solely at me. This was not the death that overtook the elderly and the infirm; this Death was strong and powerful, engaged in a struggle with me to wrest my very lifeblood, my eldest son. I recoiled from the pounding pulse of the music until it gradually faded; this time the song's ending notes left me only with darkness.

I didn't know when I got off the train whether my son would be alive or dead; it was now only a taxi ride to the truth. I smiled bitterly in the back seat of the cab as I remembered the essay by Lewis Thomas. Death had come to me on that desperate train ride home, and I had seen beyond the scientific rhetoric used to soften its countenance. This time I heard Death, and the song would never sound the same again.

Moments of Love

David S. Pisetsky, MD, PhD

When I first saw her, she was walking across the med school quad. I stood motionless as if stunned, tracking her with my eyes as she entered the classroom building. She is the one, I said to myself. It was the first day of school. When I asked a classmate about her, he told me to forget it. She's already engaged, he said. I consoled myself by concluding that she probably wasn't really right for me and that a mixer or blind date would miraculously produce a more appropriate mate.

A few months later I heard that her engagement was off, but I waited almost half a year to ask her for a date. When I telephoned her dormitory and asked nervously for her, I transposed the syllables of her first and last names into ludicrous garble. "Dinner on Saturday?" I asked tentatively, still embarrassed, expecting rejection. "I would enjoy that," she answered, sounding genuinely pleased. For the next five days my mind was locked on the thought of her as the lectures I attended compressed into senseless sound and I could envision failed examinations.

On Saturday, I greeted her at her dorm and, for the first of countless times thereafter, was entranced by her loveliness. I had made reservations at a restaurant recommended by my anatomy preceptor. Mona's was located 30 miles away at the junction where the suburbs transform into an unpredictable flux of dense forest and open field. I lost my way and drove aimlessly on rural roads for an hour, as my exasperation mounted and our conversation dwindled. She remained good-humored, happy, she said, to tour villages whose histories she had read.

We never located the restaurant and then almost ran out of gas, the search for a service station nearly as futile as the search for the restaurant. We finally ate at 10 PM at a diner near the highway, feasting on hamburgers and fries. In her floral party dress, with her straight blond hair and classic features, she stood out among the local kids, who wore hippie clothes and vacant expressions.

When we returned to the city, I was ready to apologize for the evening. As we walked from my car—a dented VW with a "Stop the War" sticker—I felt her warm hand take mine, and then, at the dormitory steps, she quickly kissed my cheek. "Thank you for a wonderful evening," she said softly. Before I comprehended what had happened, she disappeared into the building.

How many times have there been moments like that, moments of such encompassing grace and love that I doubted their actuality? If I were a man in whom religion instead of science had taken hold, I would have offered thanks, praying that these moments were real and not the dreams they sometimes seemed.

Moments like the day of our marriage, when on a crisp Sunday morning on the Pacific coast she entered the church on her father's arm and I gazed down the aisle at my soon-to-be wife. I could hear the joyful murmurs rise from the guests, captivated at her sight, and I realized that the ornate hairdo I had so strenuously objected to made her look even more appealing.

Or the moments when our children were born. In an instant her face became radiant as she emerged from the unreachable trance of labor into exultation. I furiously clicked my camera as if photographs could retain better than memory the splendor of the events and the force of those feelings.

Or the moments when she waved to me as I entered the auditorium of our children's school to watch them perform in plays or receive scholastic prizes. She would be sitting in the front row, having rearranged her morning schedule to arrive early and guarantee us good seats. I would race in from the hospital, breathless and barely on time. She would sit straight and composed, although I knew that inside she was giddy with excitement and pride.

But September 23, 1993, was different. That day, we arose at 5 AM, having hardly slept. How can you rest when a blade will soon sever flesh so dear? She kissed each of our children as they slept, but they never stirred or said "Good luck" or "I love you, Mommy."

As we drove to the hospital, our conversation was controlled and purposely trivial as we reviewed the after-school schedule for our children's practices and lessons and the car pool arrangements I would handle. "And don't forget to water the plants on Thursday. That's also the day for recycling," she said earnestly as we pulled into the hospital parking lot. I told her I had everything under control and that if I had any questions I would consult the list of instructions she had so thoughtfully typed.

In the hospital, after we signed the papers, she handed me her wedding ring for safekeeping and exchanged a gold bracelet, my gift for our fifth wedding anniversary, for a plastic band with her patient number and blood type. Then, in a barren room painted an unobtrusive green, I watched her change into a faded cotton gown and two pairs of socks, as if the worst injury that day would be the chill of the operating room.

She cried in my arms and said she didn't want the surgery. I held her hand as an IV was inserted and a cheerful nurse pressed a syringe and shimmering liquid passed through a translucent tube into her arm. In a few seconds her tears stopped and she closed those eyes that had always seemed so clever and clear but now looked so fearful. Her words slurred and a calm settled upon her, and I thought she smiled.

I felt as if the medicine flowed from her body into mine, but in me the effect was paradoxical. I felt frantic and disconnected as I watched her slow breathing. I kissed her cheek, now lax from the sedative, and then an aide with large muscles and a detached look came to help the nurse transfer her to a gurney. They pushed her away from me, down the hall and through the unforgiving doors of the operating suite.

I took the elevator to the ward where she would stay and spent the day in the waiting room drinking hospital coffee dispensed by a volunteer who hovered with concern and reminded me of one of the relatives I had met at our wedding. The coffee tasted chemical and burned, but I downed it ardently as I caught up on paperwork that had eluded me in the preceding weeks. I fiddled with the trackball on my laptop computer as I polished a manuscript whose only significance was its power to distract.

When she was returned to her room late that afternoon, on her chest was an expanse of billowing white bandage placed by a surgeon's hands with a precision and delicacy she would have admired. I was reminded of the coverlet she had appliquéd for our children's cradle when they were infants and slept at the foot of our bed. The bandage looked gentle and protective, reassuring and not as harsh as I had expected.

Sitting beside her in a dimly lit room that smelled sharply of disinfectant, I realized that because my life was so intertwined with hers, I too was a patient. I felt depleted and wrecked as I stared blankly out the window as pink-gray clouds slowly traversed the afternoon sky.

It was almost 7 PM before she stirred. I heard her moan, then I moved to the edge of the bed as her limbs fought against the confines of her blankets. She coughed twice, making faint, fitful sounds pitched like a child's cry.

Her mouth was dry, and I lightly touched her lips with an ice chip retrieved from the pitcher on her bedside table. I brushed the gray-flecked hair across her sweaty brow.

"I love you," I said.

At these words, her eyes opened hesitantly. At first her gaze seemed confused and unfocused, but for an instant her eyes sharpened with recognition, and a gentle smile lifted the edges of her mouth.

"I love you too," she whispered drowsily. Her eyelids fluttered closed as she lapsed again into the thrall of sedative sleep.

I was close to exhaustion and dislocated in time as I recalled the moment I first saw her. It was as if I was young again and the sun was resplendent in the morning sky. She is the one, I said once again in my mind's voice. She is the one.

For Everything a Blessing

Kenneth M. Prager, MD

When I was an elementary school student in Yeshiva—a Jewish parochial school with both religious and secular studies—my classmates and I used to find amusing a sign that was posted just outside the bathroom. It was an ancient Jewish blessing, commonly referred to as the *asher yatzar* benediction, that was supposed to be recited after one relieved oneself. For grade school children, there could be nothing more strange or ridiculous than to link the acts of micturition and defecation with holy words that mentioned God's name. Blessings were reserved for prayers, for holy days, or for thanking God for food or for some act of deliverance, but surely not for a bodily function that evoked smirks and giggles.

It took me several decades to realize the wisdom that lay behind this blessing that was composed by Abayei, a fourth-century Babylonian rabbi.

Abayei's blessing is contained in the Talmud, an encyclopedic work of Jewish law and lore that was written over the first five centuries of the common era. The Jewish religion is chock-full of these blessings, or *brachot*, as they are called in Hebrew. In fact, an entire tractate of Talmud, 128 pages in length, is devoted to *brachot*.

On page 120 (*Brachot* 60b) of the ancient text it is written: "Abayei said, when one comes out of a privy he should say: Blessed is He who has formed man in wisdom and created in him many orifices and many cavities. It is obvious and known before Your throne of glory that if one of them were to be ruptured or one of them blocked, it would be impossible for a man to survive and stand before You. Blessed are You that heals all flesh and does wonders."

An observant Jew is supposed to recite this blessing in Hebrew after each visit to the bathroom. We young Yeshiva students were reminded of our obligation to recite this prayer by the signs that contained its text that were posted just outside the rest room doors.

It is one thing, however, to post these signs and it is quite another to realistically expect preadolescents to have the maturity to realize the wisdom of and need for reciting a 1600-year-old blessing related to bodily functions.

It was not until my second year of medical school that I first began to understand the appropriateness of this short prayer. Pathophysiology brought home to me the terrible consequences of even minor aberrations in the structure and function of the human body. At the very least, I began to no longer take for granted the normalcy of my trips to the bathroom. Instead, I started to realize how many things had to operate just right for these minor interruptions of my daily routine to run smoothly.

I thought of Abayei and his blessing. I recalled my days at Yeshiva and remembered how silly that sign outside the bathroom had seemed. But after seeing patients whose lives revolved around their dialysis machines, and others with colostomies and urinary catheters, I realized how wise the rabbi had been.

And then it happened: I began to recite Abayei's *bracha*. At first I had to go back to my *siddur*, the Jewish prayer book, to get the text right. With repetition—and there were many opportunities for a novice to get to know this blessing well—I could recite it fluently and with sincerity and understanding.

Over the years, reciting the *asher yatzar* has become for me an opportunity to offer thanks not just for the proper functioning of my excretory organs, but for my overall good health. The text, after all, refers to catastrophic consequences of the rupture or obstruction of any bodily structure, not only those of the urinary or gastrointestinal tract. Could Abayei, for example, have foreseen that "blockage" of the "cavity," or lumen, of the coronary artery would lead to the commonest cause of death in industrialized countries some 16 centuries later?

I have often wondered if other people also yearn for some way to express gratitude for their good health. Physicians especially, who are exposed daily to the ravages that illness can wreak, must sometimes feel the need to express thanks for being well and thus well-being. Perhaps a generic, non-denominational *asher yatzar* could be composed for those who want to verbalize their gratitude for being blessed with good health.

There was one unforgettable patient whose story reinforced the truth and beauty of the *asher yatzer* for me forever. Josh was a 20-year-old student who sustained an unstable fracture of his third and fourth cervical vertebrae in a motor vehicle crash. He nearly died from his injury and required emergency intubation and ventilatory support. He was initially totally quadriplegic but for weak flexion of his right biceps.

A long and difficult period of stabilization and rehabilitation followed. There were promising signs of neurological recovery over the first few months that came suddenly and unexpectedly: movement of a finger here, flexion of a toe there, return of sensation here, adduction of a muscle group there. With incredible courage, hard work, and an excellent physical therapist, Josh improved day by day. In time, and after what seemed like a miracle, he was able to walk slowly with a leg brace and a cane.

But Josh continued to require intermittent catheterization. I knew only too well the problems and perils this young man would face for the rest of his life because of a neurogenic bladder. The urologists were very pessimistic about his chances for not requiring catheterization. They had not seen this occur after a spinal cord injury of this severity.

Then the impossible happened. I was there the day Josh no longer required a urinary catheter. I thought of Abayei's *asher yatzar* prayer. Pointing out that I could not imagine a more meaningful scenario for its recitation, I suggested to Josh, who was also a Yeshiva graduate, that he say the prayer. He agreed. As he recited the ancient *bracha*, tears welled in my eyes.

Josh is my son.

A Conversation With My Mother

David M. Eddy, MD, PhD

You have already met my father.[1] Now meet my mother. She died a few weeks ago. She wanted me to tell you how.

Her name was Virginia. Up until about six months ago, at age 84, she was the proverbial "little old lady in sneakers." After my father died of colon cancer several years ago, she lived by herself in one of those grand old Greek revival houses you see on postcards of small New England towns. Hers was in Middlebury, Vermont.

My mother was very independent, very self-sufficient, and very content. My brother and his family lived next door. Although she was quite close to them, she tried hard not to interfere in their lives. She spent most of her time reading large-print books, working word puzzles, and watching the news and professional sports on TV. She liked the house kept full of light. Every day she would take two outings, one in the morning to the small country store across the street to pick up the *Boston Globe*, and one in the afternoon to the Grand Union across town, to pick up some item she purposefully omitted from the previous day's shopping list. She did this in all but the worst weather. On icy days, she would wear golf shoes to keep from slipping and attach spikes to the tip of her cane. I think she was about 5 feet 2 and 120 pounds, but I am not certain. I know she started out at about 5 feet 4, but she seemed to shrink a little bit each year, getting cuter with time as many old people do. Her wrinkles matched her age, emphasizing a permanent thin-lipped smile that extended all the way to her little Kris Kringle eyes. The only thing that embarrassed her was her thinning gray hair, but she covered that up with a rather dashing tweed fedora that matched her Talbots outfits. She loved to tease people by wearing outrageous necklaces. The one made from the front teeth of camels was her favorite.

To be sure, she had had her share of problems in the past: diverticulitis and endometriosis when she was younger, more recently a broken hip, a bout with depression, some hearing loss, and cataracts. But she was a walking tribute to the best things in American medicine. Coming from a family of four generations of physicians, she was fond of bragging that, but for lens implants, hearing aids, hip surgery, and Elavil, she would be blind, deaf, bedridden, and depressed. At age 84, her only problems were a slight rectal prolapse, which she could reduce fairly easily, some urinary incontinence, and a fear that if her eyesight got much worse she would lose her main pleasures. But those things were easy to deal with and she was, to use her New England expression, "happy as a clam."

"David, I can't tell you how content I am. Except for missing your father, these are the best years of my life."

Yes, all was well with my mother, until about six months ago. That was when she developed acute cholelithiasis. From that point on, her health began to unravel with amazing speed. She recovered from the cholecystectomy on schedule and within a few weeks of leaving the hospital was resuming her walks downtown. But about six weeks after the surgery she was suddenly hit with a case of severe diarrhea, so severe that it extended her rectal prolapse to about eight inches and dehydrated her to the point that she had to be readmitted. As soon as her physician got her rehydrated, other complications quickly set in. She developed oral thrush, apparently due to the antibiotic treatment for her diarrhea, and her antidepressants got out of balance. For some reason that was never fully determined, she also became anemic, which was treated with iron, which made her nauseated. She could not eat, she got weak, her skin itched, and her body ached. Oh yes, they also found a lump in her breast, the diagnosis of which was postponed, and atrial fibrillation. Needless to say, she was quite depressed.

Her depression was accentuated by the need to deal with her rectal prolapse. On the one hand, she really disliked the thought of more surgery. She especially hated the nasogastric tube and the intense postoperative fatigue. On the other hand, the prolapse was very painful. The least cough or strain would send it out to rub against the sheets, and she could not push it back the way she used to. She knew that she could not possibly walk to the Grand Union again unless it was fixed.

It was at that time that she first began to talk to me about how she could end her life gracefully. As a physician's wife, she was used to thinking about life and death and prided herself on being able to deal maturely with the idea of death. She had signed every living will and advance directive she could find, and carried a card that donated her organs. Even though she knew they would not do anyone much good (*"Can they recycle my artificial hip and lenses?"*), she liked the way the card announced her acceptance of the fact that all things must someday end. She dreaded the thought of being in a nursing home, unable to take care of herself, her body, mind, and interests progressively declining until she was little more than a blank stare, waiting for death to mercifully take her away.

"I know they can keep me alive a long time, but what's the point? If the pleasure is gone and the direction is steadily down, why should I have to draw it out until I'm 'rescued' by cancer, a heart attack, or a stroke? That could take years. I understand that some people want to hang on until all the possible treatments have been tried to squeeze out the last drops of life. That's fine for them. But not for me."

My own philosophy, undoubtedly influenced heavily by my parents, is that choosing the best way to end your life should be the ultimate individual right—a right to be exercised between oneself and one's beliefs, without intrusions from governments or the beliefs of others. On the other hand, I also believe that such decisions should be made only with an accurate understanding of one's prognosis and should never be made in the middle of a correctable depression or a temporary trough. So my brother, sister, and I coaxed her to see a rectal surgeon about having her prolapse repaired and to put off thoughts of suicide until her health problems were stabilized and her antidepressants were back in balance.

With the surgeon's help, we explored the possible outcomes of the available procedures for her prolapse. My mother did not mind the higher mortality rates of the more extensive operations—in fact, she wanted them. Her main concern was to avoid rectal incontinence, which she knew would dampen any hopes of returning to her former lifestyle.

Unfortunately, that was the outcome she got. By the time she had recovered from the rectal surgery, she was totally incontinent "at both ends," to use her words. She was bedridden, anemic, exhausted, nauseated, achy, and itchy. Furthermore, over the period of this illness her eyesight had begun to fail to the point she could no longer read. Because she was too sick to live at home, even with my brother's help, but not sick enough to be hospitalized, we had to move her to an intermediate care facility.

On the positive side, her antidepressants were working again and she had regained her clarity of mind, her spirit, and her humor. But she was very unhappy. She knew instinctively, and her physician confirmed, that after all the insults of the past few months it was very unlikely she would ever be able to take care of herself alone or walk to the Grand Union. That was when she began to press me harder about suicide.

"Let me put this in terms you should understand, David. My 'quality of life'—isn't that what you call it?—has dropped below zero. I know there is nothing fatally wrong with me and that I could live on for many more years. With a colostomy and some luck I might even be able to recover a bit of my former lifestyle, for a while. But do we have to do that just because it's possible? Is the meaning of life defined by its duration? Or does life have a purpose so large that it doesn't have to be prolonged at any cost to preserve its meaning?

"I've lived a wonderful life, but it has to end sometime and this is the right time for me. My decision is not about whether I'm going to die—we will all die sooner or later. My decision is about when and how. I don't want to spoil the wonder of my life by dragging it out in years of decay. I want to go now, while the good memories are still fresh. I have always known that eventually the right time would come, and now I know that this is it. Help me find a way."

I discussed her request with my brother and sister and with her nurses and physician. Although we all had different feelings about her request, we agreed that she satisfied our criteria of being well-informed, stable, and not depressed. For selfish reasons we wanted her to live as long as possible, but we realized that it was not our desires that mattered. What mattered to us were her wishes. She was totally rational about her conviction that this was "her time." Now she was asking for our help, and it struck us as the height of paternalism (or filialism?) to impose our desires over hers.

I bought *Final Exit*[2] for her, and we read it together. If she were to end her life, she would obviously have to do it with pills. But as anyone who has thought about this knows, accomplishing that is not easy. Patients can rarely get the pills themselves, especially in a controlled setting like a hospital or nursing home. Anyone who provides the pills knowing they will be used for suicide could be arrested. Even if those problems are solved and the pills are available, they can be difficult to take, especially by the frail. Most likely, my mother would fall asleep before she could swallow the full dose. A way around this would be for her to put a bag over her head with a rubber band at her neck to ensure that she would suffocate if she fell asleep before taking all the pills. But my mother did not like that idea because of the depressing picture it would present to those who found her body. She contemplated drawing a happy smile on the bag, but did not think that would give the correct impression either. The picture my mother wanted to leave to the world was that her death was a happy moment, like the end of a wonderful movie, a time for good memories and a peaceful acceptance of whatever the future might hold. She did not like the image of being a quasi-criminal sneaking illegal medicines. The way she really wanted to die was to be given a morphine drip that she could control, to have her family around her holding her hands, and for her to turn up the drip.

As wonderful as that might sound, it is illegal. One problem was that my mother did not have a terminal condition or agonizing pain that might justify a morphine drip. Far from it. Her heart was strong enough to keep her alive for ten more years, albeit as a frail, bedridden, partially blind, partially deaf, incontinent, and possibly stroked-out woman. But beyond that, no physician would dare give a patient access to a lethal medicine in a way that could be accused of assisting suicide. Legally, physicians can provide lots of comfort care, even if it might hasten a patient's death, but the primary purpose of the medicine must be to relieve suffering, not to cause death. Every now and then my mother would vent her frustration with the law and the arrogance of others who insist that everyone must accept their philosophy of death, but she knew that railing at what she considered to be misguided laws would not undo them. She needed to focus on finding a solution to her problem. She decided that the only realistic way out was for me to get her some drugs and for her to do her best to swallow them. Although I was very nervous at the thought of being turned in by someone who discovered our plan and felt it was their duty to stop it, I was willing to do my part. I respected her decision, and I knew she would do the same for me.

I had no difficulty finding a friend who could write a prescription for restricted drugs and who was willing to help us from a distance. In fact, I have yet to find anybody who agrees with the current laws. (*"So why do they exist?"*) But before I actually had to resolve any lingering conflicts and obtain the drugs, my mother's course took an unexpected and strangely welcomed twist. I received a call that she had developed pneumonia and had to be readmitted to the hospital. By the time I made contact with her, she had already reminded her attendants that she did not want to be resuscitated if she should have a heart attack or stroke.

"Is there anything more I can do?"

Pneumonia, the old folks' friend, I thought to myself. I told her that although advance directives usually apply to refusing treatments for emergencies such as heart attacks, it was always legal for her to refuse any treatment. In particular, she could refuse the antibiotics for the pneumonia. Her physician and nurses would undoubtedly advise her against it, but if she signed enough papers they would have to honor her request.

"What's it like to die of pneumonia? Will they keep me comfortable?"

I knew that without any medicine for comfort, pneumonia was not a pleasant way to die. But I was also confident that her physician was compassionate and would keep her comfortable. So she asked that the antibiotics be stopped. Given the deep gurgling in her throat every time she breathed, we all expected the infection to spread rapidly. She took a perverse pleasure in that week's cover story of *Newsweek*, which described the spread of resistant strains.

"Bring all the resistant strains in this hospital to me. That will be my present to the other patients."

But that did not happen. Against the odds, her pneumonia regressed. This discouraged her greatly—to see the solution so close, just to watch it slip away.

"What else can I do? Can I stop eating?"

I told her she could, but that that approach could take a long time. I then told her that if she was really intent on dying, she could stop drinking. Without water, no one, even the healthiest, can live more than a few days.

"Can they keep me comfortable?"

I talked with her physician. Although it ran against his instincts, he respected the clarity and firmness of my mother's decision and agreed that her quality of life had sunk below what she was willing to bear. He also knew that what she was asking from him was legal. He took out the IV and wrote orders that she should receive adequate medications to control discomfort.

My mother was elated. The next day happened to be her 85th birthday, which we celebrated with a party, balloons and all. She was beaming from ear to ear. She had done it. She had found the way. She relished her last piece of chocolate, and then stopped eating and drinking.

Over the next four days, my mother greeted her visitors with the first smiles she had shown for months. She energetically reminisced about the great times she had had and about things she was proud of. (She especially hoped I would tell you about her traveling alone across Africa at the age of

70, and surviving a capsized raft on Wyoming's Snake River at 82.) She also found a calming self-acceptance in describing things of which she was not proud. She slept between visits but woke up brightly whenever we touched her to share more memories and say a few more things she wanted us to know. On the fifth day it was more difficult to wake her. When we would take her hand she would open her eyes and smile, but she was too drowsy and weak to talk very much. On the sixth day, we could not wake her. Her face was relaxed in her natural smile, she was breathing unevenly, but peacefully. We held her hands for another two hours, until she died.

I had always imagined that when I finally stood in the middle of my parents' empty house, surrounded by the old smells, by hundreds of objects that represent a time forever lost, and by the terminal silence, I would be overwhelmingly saddened. But I wasn't. This death was not a sad death; it was a happy death. It did not come after years of decline, lost vitality, and loneliness; it came at the right time. My mother was not clinging desperately to what no one can have. She knew that death was not a tragedy to be postponed at any cost, but that death is a part of life, to be embraced at the proper time. She had done just what she wanted to do, just the way she wanted to do it. Without hoarding pills, without making me a criminal, without putting a bag over her head, and without huddling in a van with a carbon monoxide machine, she had found a way to bring her life gracefully to a close. Of course we cried. But although we will miss her greatly, her ability to achieve her death at her "right time" and in her "right way" transformed for us what could have been a desolate and crushing loss into a time for joy. Because she was happy, we were happy.

"Write about this, David. Tell others how well this worked for me. I'd like this to be my gift. Whether they are terminally ill, in intractable pain, or, like me, just know that the right time has come for them, more people might want to know that this way exists. And maybe more physicians will help them find it."

Maybe they will. Rest in peace, Mom.

My mother wants to thank Dr Timothy Cope of Middlebury, Vermont, for his present on her 85th birthday.

1. Eddy DM. Cost-effectiveness analysis: a conversation with my father. *JAMA*. 1992;267:1669-1672, 1674-1675.
2. Humphry D. *Final Exit*. Secaucus, NJ: Carol Publishing Group; 1991.

The Dark Side

Most physicians have been exposed to violence at some point in their careers: treating survivors of domestic abuse or criminal assault in the emergency department or office, or experiencing it themselves. How do they cope? In "First Encounter," a medical student witnesses firsthand a fatal shooting and vows, perhaps naively, that he will never let Death get the better of him. In the moving and mind-boggling "Belinda, Asleep Without Dreams," a forensic pathologist helplessly observes the grim result of a heinous act of violence against a 13-month-old child who will be disconnected from life support after the pathologist gathers evidence. (The author telephoned me several years after publication of the essay to inform me—with grim satisfaction, which I shared—that the perpetrator had been convicted of the crime and sentenced to prison.) Whether witnessing the horrifying effects of war ("The Messengers") or, worse, becoming a gun-user himself after learning of the death of his friend ("Frozen in Time"), these authors have seen the worst atrocities that a person can commit against another, often for little or no reason. Remarkably, the experiences may have made these physicians better people because of it.

R.K.Y.

Do Angels Cry?

Matko Marušić, MD, PhD

Do not cry," the guardian angel said to Goran. "Angels do not cry."

"I have to cry. My father is crying for me, and nobody can help him," replied Goran. "Everyone is just standing and weeping. Why is nobody trying to comfort him?"

Goran saw his father, his body twisting with pain, some people standing around and Jurica lying a little farther away. His father's hopeless tears were not so much from grief but from fear and from disbelief that Goran was killed and that he lay before him both dead and warm, his face pale, his body outstretched, as though he was pretending to sleep.

"Help my father, stop him from crying, comfort him," Goran pleaded with the invisible angel who stood behind him.

"I cannot. I am your guardian angel. I am forbidden to help other people," the angel replied softly and sadly.

"Why did you not save me then?" Goran rebuked, not on account of himself but on account of his father.

"I could not save you," the angel replied. "That is in the hands of our Lord. I spared you from pain. That is all I could do."

Indeed, Goran had died quickly and painlessly, in a single moment, without fear, or disfigurement. The bomb could not reach him in the shelter, but it had caused a dreadful shock wave that killed him and Jurica, his friend. They neither heard nor saw the explosion; they just lost their breath and died. The demolished house toppled in on the shelter, but their little bodies were untouched; they remained in the corner of the room between the roof that had fallen and the walls that were still standing; pale and tender, innocent and gentle, their bodies unscarred, just a little blood on their ears. Their guardian angels held up the roof so it did not maim them, tenderly closed their eyelids, wiped the blood from their ears, and led them to God. They saw His face and were happy to be accepted among the angels. Still, when they sat at the right hand of God, Goran saw his father below, digging through the rubble for his body, and was no longer happy.

Goran knew his father well: there was nothing he was afraid of and he always kept his feelings to himself. He was bent on making life easier and nicer for his children. He spoke little and was stern looking, but everyone knew that he was gentle. When Goran's brother Ante died fighting at the front lines, his father did not cry. Goran did not see the body. Only his father went to see him at the hospital; he brought back Ante's shirt. Their mother washed the shirt, but his father did not let her mend it. And he did not cry. He drank, but he did not cry. He talked with people about how Ante was brave. But now he cried for Goran, perhaps because Goran was young and innocent, unable to harm anyone, and nobody had a reason or a need to kill him. And Goran began to cry.

"Don't cry, angels don't cry," the guardian angel repeated. "Now you will also guard someone and you must be serious and collect yourself."

"I want to guard my father, I wish he would stop crying, my father never cries. This is upsetting me!" replied Goran, wiping his own tears.

"No, angels can only guard innocent children. Your father is an adult and a warrior. We are not allowed to guard warriors," advised the guardian angel.

"Please, just so he would stop crying!" pleaded Goran, but the angel remained silent and could only tenderly caress his shoulder.

At the beginning his father did not cry. With two friends he cleared the shelter, pulling at beams and bars with his strong hands. From beneath the rubble nothing could be heard, and he was frightened for his son, but he kept digging. Finally, the room was cleared and he saw that Goran was dead. He cried without tears, frightened and with despair, perhaps wanting to believe that it was untrue. The men pulled him away and continued to dig. Nobody tried to comfort him. When a warrior cries for his son nobody can comfort him. He watched, not knowing he was crying. He continued to cry when they took Goran and Jurica from the shelter and laid their bodies on the lawn and covered them to the shoulders. He cried for Jurica too, but for Goran he could not cry enough. Men stood by silently, their heads bowed, like at prayer. He crouched by Goran and called out to him. But Goran lay silent and pale, with the same hair, with the same face, untouched and small, as though he was asleep and about to rise.

"Help him, Lord. Help him, my guardian angel," cried Goran in the heavens, but there was no answer. The angel's hand squeezed his shoulder tighter.

His father caressed his face and hair. Knowing he was dead, his father continued to caress him as though he were alive, as Goran had liked this the most. And as he stroked him it seemed that Goran was still alive. Nobody spoke. Beside Jurica stood men with bowed heads. Jurica's father was not there. He was at the fighting.

"Let us pray for Jurica," the guardian angel remembered, and they prayed together with Jurica and his guardian angel, with bright angelic voices that bring comfort. Goran stopped crying.

At that moment, his father knelt beside Goran and hugged his soft body. He felt his thin ribs and small shoulders, just as he always had before Goran went to sleep. Goran's body was still warm. His father kissed his cheeks, but they were cold. It was then that he saw the traces of blood beside his ears and realized that he could not help. His tears were no longer frightened but hopeless and desperate. He did not know that Goran worriedly watched him from the heavens.

"Don't cry, Goran, don't cry," said the guardian angel in a faltering voice. "You shall find one another in the hands of God. Death cannot do anything to righteous people; and the suffering of those on Earth. . . ."

It was then that his angelic voice broke, and he cried with greater bitterness than Goran had. He hugged the boy with his strong, unseen arms and also kissed his white face. They cried openly and inconsolably as Goran's father was hugging and kissing his son's white face.

"Angels cry too," thought Goran, and the guardian angel heard and said:

"Angels cry the most, Goran, because angels guard children, and it is the most sorrowful when a child dies."

Lord had seen and heard all, but He said nothing. We do not know what He thought, what He wished, and whether He had cried. God works in mysterious ways, but only He can carry the weight of sadness for Goran and Jurica, children who were killed in Slavonski Brod, His day the June 24, 1992.

Translated by S. Jureta and V. Kabalin.

The Messengers

LTC Michael V. Slayter, VC, USA

It was the hairpin that caught my eye. In its grasp, the strands of hair were not guided to any particular style; no, more a matter of convenience. It was off-center and appeared to have been put on hurriedly, perhaps just before bedtime.

———

The large doors opened as the gigantic refrigerator truck backed up to the opening of the building, its rear panel agape with two large marines standing on either side. The truck stopped even with the edge of the building, blocking out the winter light that was causing us to shade our eyes. Our vision adjusted, and we saw the aluminum cases, 28 of them, stacked to the ceiling of the truck's interior. The C-5 jet transport that had brought them from Saudi Arabia to Dover Air Force Base was still on the parking ramp about a mile away. As the crowd of military volunteers formed two lines of body handlers, the cases were guided off the truck and snapped open. Heavy zippers made a ripping sound under gloved hands, and 28 Americans found their way back home. We stood transfixed at seeing what a madman with a Scud missile could do, even in the final hours of a war. What had been only a news item on television was now a reality at our fingertips. They were rear echelon troops. The "safe" ones.

Before preparation for their return to their families, protocol requires that the record of each casualty contain a description of all wounds and a medical statement regarding cause of death. I was conscripted into assisting the medical examiner's team with this part of the task, the last step before embalming. In a way, I was glad that I had made two previous trips to Dover and caught a glimpse of the activities and procedures there. The most casualties I had seen at one time were two or possibly three over the span of a day. Each time I witnessed the primary business of this solemn place, I would instinctively try to assume the objective, professional attitude of those around me. I suppose anyone would do that. Don't let it show . . . that's not why we're here . . . plenty of folks to mourn back home. We are at war; certain losses are said to be acceptable.

But the hairpin ripped a hole in my objectivity; ripped it and made it bleed. The pin was imperfectly placed, but with a definite purpose; perhaps with a small touch of pride. It was placed there by someone who felt something; felt the need for sleep; felt the anticipation of a night's rest; longed for home; wondered about tomorrow. . . . I had helped document four individuals when I stopped for a short break and saw this small messenger in her hair only a few feet away on the next table, pulling at me like a magnet. Suddenly, all I cared about was returning to my previous state of mind, where emotions were not always welcome, where the soul was insulated from hurt. I must have been doing well at first, because I barely remember those first four cases, but the next three will stay with me for a long time. Returning to my work table, I began to see every small wrinkle, every line, every detail of each one. Eyes . . . they all had eyes; I know, because I had been recording their descriptions. But now I saw all the tiny variations in color that I was certain only a mother would notice. Haircuts, scars, blemishes, a tattoo all began to surround me, shouting and proclaiming their owners' uniqueness. Hardest of all was realizing the tenderness of their years, so close to that of my own two children. Had they ever been in love? Were they admired by others? Would anyone at home miss them?

At last by midafternoon we were done, and I vaguely remember saying good-bye to my coworkers as I left. Why did the walk from the building to the parking lot seem so much longer than it had that morning? It was cold, and the February wind bit at my face. I reached my car, unlocked the door, and gazed back at the building where I had just left a small scrap of my own soul; it now seemed a world away. As I began to drive away, another huge jet lumbered overhead, engines whining, the air cupped under its monstrous wings. Having seen the incoming flight schedule, I knew this plane carried only inanimate cargo. In my numbness, I almost forgot to slow down at the exit to the base, giving the young guard a moment's hesitation and confusion before he snapped a salute.

I drove a few miles before realizing I hadn't yet eaten lunch. Surprisingly, I wasn't hungry; or maybe it didn't surprise me. Gradually, I felt myself trying to summarize the day. I couldn't escape the crazy notion that I was missing something: a message, a revelation, something magical. I pulled over and stopped, then went over each case in my mind, one by one, trying mostly to remember details of the first four. As the seconds ticked by, other mundane thoughts seeped in, and the drama back at Dover seemed to separate from me. As I swung back onto the highway, I felt the knot in my stomach loosen and disappear. After all, the war was over. Don't make this into something it isn't, I thought.

Two hours later and back at my office in Washington, DC, I must have seemed quietly cavalier about the whole event. The best comment I could utter was to express thanks the war was over. How noble, how aloof! I'd just witnessed more death than most people see in a lifetime, and I heroically chose to focus only on the big picture! I carried that strong, silent demeanor home with me that evening, but my defensive wall felt a small tremor when my two teenaged sons greeted me at the door. How quickly the mind repairs walls.

I went through that evening and the next day as usual, my thoughts and movements focused on the pile of work on my desk. That evening my wife and I, along with some neighbors, attended a concert at the high school, an event that is always fun, especially if you know the kids in the band. The first few minutes of music were lively and stirring, something one might hear during half-time at a football game. Then the director announced it was time for some soft, easy-listening numbers featuring the wind instrument section.

As the youngsters turned the pages on their music stands, a tall, slender girl in the front laid her flute in her lap and from somewhere produced a small object that I couldn't quite make out. I watched her hand go to her mouth, make a quick, almost imperceptible snapping motion; and while brushing her hair aside with the other hand, she pushed the now clearly visible hairpin into place. The earlier lively music had relaxed my invisible wall and now this slip of a girl had caught me off guard and, in an instant, took me back to Dover. As the soft notes began to flow, the pain eased for a moment. Then as I heard a heavenly solo from this little emissary with the flute, I felt the inner weeping awaken again, pulling at me, trying to wrestle my control away. How long had it been? A day and a half? Her music came as soothing notes that flowed ever so tenderly from her instrument, but firmly demanded to be heard with an overwhelming strength the likes of which I had never felt before. Her fellow musicians answered with a harmony that painted a formless picture. Formless, but with the unmistakable intent of speaking from the heart. The melody filled my ears, my head, my very being, and I wanted it to end; to have a flaw; a childish squawk or honk that would break the strain. But listening closely only brought mild fluctuations to my ears, which made it all the more perfect. Silently trapped, all I could do was focus on this young girl with the hairpin . . . placed so casually, not to any particular style; no, more a matter of convenience. It was off-center and appeared to have been put on hurriedly, as though just before bedtime.

Remembered Pain

Robert S. McKelvey, MD

I was recently called to consult on a severely depressed, middle-aged Vietnam veteran. The resident on the case wondered aloud if the man's symptomatology—anxiety, depression, and recurrent terrifying nightmares of combat—could really be related to events of long ago. Would not time have healed his wounds? As I tried to explain to her the timelessness of emotional pain that has not been well integrated into one's experience, a memory suddenly thrust itself on me.

It was Easter Sunday—cold, overcast, and rainy—an Easter Sunday 18 years ago northwest of Da Nang in what was then South Vietnam. I was in church, my spirits buoyed by the beauty and hope of Easter music and the realization that I would soon be going home. My thoughts were interrupted by a touch on my shoulder and a whispered voice: "Captain, there's been an accident in the village. The C.O. wants you to go take a look."

On this same Easter Sunday a Vietnamese family in the village next to our base had been eating breakfast together: a man, a woman, and two young children. Suddenly, without warning except for its final, sickening scream, a mortar round impacted their patio not five feet away. The husband was killed instantly. The wife, badly wounded, would die in a few minutes. The two children, shocked and terrified by the huge explosion, have wounds that will maim but not kill them. Easter Sunday. A neighboring infantry company patrolling the Da Nang perimeter thought it detected movement. Probing rounds were fired from its 60-millimeter mortar. Somehow, one fell far short. Two Vietnamese are dead or dying, but not "the bad guys." Simple people, a farmer and his wife.

When I arrive, the area around the hut is swarming with people from the village. A Medivac helicopter is lifting off, carrying what remains of the family to a hospital in Da Nang. There is really nothing for me to do. An investigation will begin tomorrow. There is no one left in the family to whom I might apologize or offer help. As I walk back toward my jeep I am scarcely aware of the young girl walking beside me, calling to me, pulling my sleeve. "Dai Uy—my father, an explosion—come quickly." What is she talking about? I know about the explosion, the family is gone, there is no one left. Insistently, she pulls on my sleeve. There has been another accident.

She rushes ahead of me, tears in her eyes, toward a rice paddy on the edge of the village. I see her run to a body along the paddy dike. The head is covered with a conical hat. As I reach her, huddled by the motionless form, she lifts the hat for me to see. There is no face, there is scarcely a head—only a blackened horrible thing that she quickly covers. I feel sick, angry, enraged that this has happened a quarter mile from another tragedy. Slowly she gasps out her story. Her father had left early that morning to work in the rice paddy. It is the time when the paddy is prepared for spring planting. Today he had wanted to shape the dike, straightening its sides, which had collapsed from the heavy rains of winter. As his hoe worked the side of the dike, rising and falling in an arc from above his head to the earth below, it struck a hidden remnant of the war. A grenade—fired from an M-79 grenade launcher—had bored into the dike, unexploded. Struck by the hoe's blade, it exploded now, ripping open his chest, tearing apart his face, and blasting away most of his head. It must have happened at about the same time the mortar round hit nearby.

Easter Sunday. Three civilians dead, killed without warning while engaged in the simple, straightforward business of their daily lives. Two new orphans, a family without a father, a little girl sobbing by a paddy dike. Where was the hope, the expectancy of Easter morning? I got into my jeep in a blind rage. I could not even answer my driver's questions. The only thought in my mind was to grab God by His lapels and shake Him. What in the hell is the meaning of this? Where are You? Why do You let this insanity go on?

As I recalled that Easter Sunday so long ago I was overcome by a profound sadness and my eyes filled with tears. Eighteen years had flown by in an instant and I was a young man again, kneeling by a little girl, crying with her. I had found the answer to the resident's question. Memory is timeless. The pain of past experience is always with us. If we have not found ways to seal it off or integrate it into our experience, it has the power to seize and overwhelm us. Would the young physician understand? She would if she looked into her own heart, into her own pain and sadness. Then she would join me on the paddy dike, beside a young girl whose world had been swept away.

Belinda, Asleep Without Dreams

Kris Sperry, MD

Visitors are few and far between in the pediatric intensive care unit at 3 AM. When I walked through the doors, the nurses clustered between the faintly beeping monitors that flanked their work area paused and turned in unison, to look at me. I identified myself, showing them my medical investigator's office badge and university ID card, and told them that the police had called and asked me to look at a little child who had been under their watchful care for only a few hours. I could not immediately remember the child's name; the telephone call 45 minutes earlier was rather hazy in my memory. When I scanned the patient roster posted on the wall, I found the right name: Belinda. Her nurse took me to the child's bedside.

Pathologists usually do not encounter problems that cannot wait until morning. For several years, though, the forensic pathologists with the medical investigator's office have been working directly with the child abuse units of both the local police department and the district attorney's office. We evaluate traumatic injuries frequently and are not as reluctant to testify in court as other physicians. This expertise has often aided in the successful prosecution of abuse cases. Thus, I found myself at Belinda's hospital bed in the middle of the night, trying to fill in some of the puzzle pieces that would help explain how she got there.

Belinda lay motionless, her small chest rising and falling slowly in time with the "chuff" sound made by the pediatric ventilator. She appeared asleep, quiet and at rest, with her delicate features marred only by the endotracheal tube taped across her mouth. Monitor wires crossed her trunk, and intravenous lines were innocuously anchored to her short, chubby arms with Velcro splints. I started my examination, carefully moving and inspecting her arms and legs. A couple of small, healing abrasions on her legs were the sole injuries, legacies of an angry kitty cat grabbed a few days ago by this curious 13-month-old toddler. No marks discolored the chest or abdomen, and the back was likewise uninjured. I turned her head this way and that, looking for anything that might help explain her deep, unarousable sleep, and found only tiny hemorrhagic cutaneous suffusions over the mastoid regions, subtly heralding internal disasters. I separated her fine, straight blond hairs, but found nothing on her scalp.

After a short journey downstairs to radiology, I located her skull films. The massive trauma revealed by the x-ray films was overwhelming: linear skull fractures coursed anteriorly over the entire length of both parietal bones, meeting posteriorly just left of midline, with sutural separations connecting the radiolucent fracture lines. Tomographic brain scans recorded extremely severe cerebral edema in shades of gray, with the black spaces that represent the ventricular spaces reduced to mere slits by the swelling.

These radiological revelations were followed by extended telephone discourses with the child abuse detectives, who were encamped at a house where, not even 12 hours before, Belinda had been under the care of a baby-sitter. During the afternoon, the sitter's husband "found" the toddler unconscious within her playpen, initiating this nightmarish sequence that was only too real. I answered the police queries: No, the injury could not have been sustained in a fall within the home, or from the playpen. Yes, the injury was directly inflicted by another individual, most probably an adult, who had slammed the back of Belinda's head down onto a hard, unyielding surface with such force that the only comparable injuries would be those seen in a head-on vehicle collision. Yes, Belinda was probably going to die, as her brain was swollen beyond the cranial cavity capacity.

Finally, I drove home, to catch a few hours' sleep before assuming the day's duties. In the early afternoon, the call came to me that underscored Belinda's prognosis: Could this child be considered an organ donor? An electroencephalogram was scheduled for tonight, and if the brain were devoid of cerebral activity, blood flow studies would follow tomorrow to inarguably prove brain death. Then, the organ harvest, followed by feverish activity to fly these precious gifts to anonymous ailing children around the country. Belinda would then come to me, where my job would be to expose, describe, and photograph the lethal injuries hinted at in the two-dimensional, colorless x-ray films I had viewed. Finally, reports would be generated, and the interminable series of discussions with attorneys would begin. And, perhaps somewhere along the line, whatever passes for justice would be served.

In the wink of an eye, an emotional outburst killed a small child, and coincidentally shattered two families just as surely as this little one's skull had been broken into jagged pieces. Guilt, recrimination, regret, and hate suddenly became paramount, fueled by suspicion. Normally placid day-to-day family activities were invaded by the legal, police, and social welfare systems, all attempting to achieve some understanding of an event that is inherently impossible to understand.

As I drove home that evening, questions raged in my thoughts: Why do we continue to kill and maim our children? What actions of a 13-month-old child are so heinous that smashing her head against the floor is the only recourse? What punishment could be meted out to the perpetrator, in the name of justice, that will even begin to replace the beauty of a single smile from this dead child? When will I never see another dead or dying baby, mortally hurt at the hands of those whom it unwaveringly loves and trusts? My heart ached, and my eyes misted over with tears of rage, frustration, and sorrow.

My own children met me at the door, eager to share their experiences in school and to show me the treasures they had constructed there. They chattered on, and I thought about what it would take for me to hurt them. I could not find an answer. Later, as they nestled against me as we read a book together, my mind crept unbidden to a small child, seemingly asleep in a hospital bed, but no longer having the dreams of warmth, security, and love that provide comfort in the dark hours of the night.

Sleep with the angels, Belinda.

A Simple Act

Reg Green

When our family—my wife Maggie, our 4-year-old Eleanor, and I—drove through Messina, Sicily, to our hotel in the early hours of the morning one day last September, I felt I had never been in a bleaker place. We didn't know a soul, the streets were deserted, and we were leaving at the hospital our 7-year-old son in a deep and dreadful coma.

We wanted only to go home, to take Nicholas with us, however badly injured, to help nurse him through whatever he faced, to hold his hand again, to put our arms around him.

It had been the worst night of our lives.

The next morning we took a bus back to the hospital. There had been no deterioration but no improvement either. "You know, there are miracles," said the man who had been appointed to act as our interpreter, but the doctors looked grave. In lives that only a few hours before had been full of warmth and laughter, there was now a gnawing emptiness.

Within days our intensely personal experience erupted into a worldwide story. Newspapers and television told of the shooting attack by car bandits, Nicholas' death, and our decision to donate his organs. Since then streets, schools, scholarships, and hospitals all over Italy have been named for him. We have received honors previously reserved largely for kings and presidents, prizes that go mainly to Nobelists and awards usually given to spiritual leaders of the stature of Mother Teresa. Maria Shriver, who all her life has been told by people where they were when President Kennedy was shot, told us where she was when she heard about Nicholas. Strangers come up to us on the street still, tears in their eyes.

We have received letters from about a thousand people around the world, written with a simple eloquence possible only when it comes straight from the heart. A 40-year-old American, who recently became blind, said our story had given him the strength to resist despair. One man who was close to death now has a new lung because someone was moved by what happened to Nicholas. A woman who lost her 4-year-old daughter imagines the two children playing happily together in a place where there is no violence.

All this for a decision that seemed so obvious we've forgotten which of us suggested it.

I remember the hushed room and the physicians standing in a small group, hesitant to ask crass questions about organ donation. As it happens, we were able to relieve them of the thankless task. We looked at each other. "Now that he's gone, shouldn't we give the organs?" one of us asked. "Yes," the other replied. And that was all there was to it.

Our decision was not clouded by any doubts about the medical staff. We were convinced they had done everything in their power to save Nicholas. To be sure, we asked how they knew his brain was truly dead, and they described their high-tech methods in clear, simple language. It helped. But more than that, it was the bond of trust that had been established from the beginning that left no doubt they would not have given up until all hope was gone.

Yet we've been asked a hundred times: How could you have done it? And a hundred times we've searched for words to convey the sense of how clear and how right the choice seemed. Nicholas was dead. He no longer looked like a sleeping child. By giving his organs we weren't hurting him but we were helping others.

For us, Nicholas will always live, in our hearts and our memories. But he wasn't in that body anymore.

His toys are still here, including the flag on his log fort, which I put at half-staff when we returned home and which has stayed that way ever since. We have assembled all his photographs, starting with the blur I snapped a few moments after he was born. Nicholas now lies in a peaceful country churchyard in California, dressed for eternity in the kind of blue blazer and neat slacks he liked and a tie with Goofy on it.

Donating his organs, then, wasn't a particularly magnanimous act. But not to have given them would have seemed to us such an act of miserliness that we don't believe we could have thought about it later without shame. The future of a radiant little creature had been taken away. It was important to us that someone else should have that future.

It turned out to be seven people's future, most of them young, most very sick. One 19-year-old within 48 hours of death ("We'd given up on her," her physician told me later) is now a vivacious beauty who turns heads as she walks down the street. The 60-pound 15-year-old who got Nicholas' heart had spent half his life in hospitals; now he's a relentless bundle of energy. One of the recipients, when told by his doctors to think of something nice as he was taken to the operating theater, said, "I am thinking of something nice. I'm thinking of Nicholas." I recently visited him at school; he's a wonderful little fellow any father would be proud of and, I admit, I did feel pride. The man who received one of Nicholas' corneas told us that at one time he was unable to see his children. Now, after two operations, he happily watches his daughter fencing and his son play rugby.

We are pleased the publicity this incident has caused should have led to such a dramatic arousal of interest in organ donation. It seems unfair, however, to the thousands of parents and children who, in lonely hospital waiting rooms around the world, have made exactly the same decision. Their loss is indistinguishable from ours, but their willingness to share rather than to hoard life has remained largely unrecognized.

I imagine that for them, like us, the emptiness is always close by. I don't believe Maggie and I will ever be really happy again; even our best moments are tinged with sadness. But our joy in seeing so much eager life that would otherwise have been lost, and the relief on the families' faces, is so uplifting that it has given us some recompense for what otherwise would have been just a sordid act of violence.

A Winter's Tale

Gregory J. Davis, MD

The long difficult week had finally come to a close, none too soon for our service. It was now early Friday evening, and an ice storm had just begun to hit with a vengeance, an unusual event for our part of the country. My customary 30-minute commute, thanks to a treacherous layer of invisible ice, had doubled.

Once home, I was greeted with my three kids' cheery "Hi, Dad!"; tantalizing smells of a chicken dinner; and the added spice of my wife Kathleen, who for a change had a Friday night off work. I stomped the slush from my shoes and hurried in, my preoccupation with the week's cases already beginning to recede. My son answered the ringing telephone and his crestfallen expression told me at once that it could only be a police officer on the other end of the line, asking for me.

As in countless evenings past, the choreography began to play itself out. Kathleen put on a fresh pot of coffee as I donned more layers of clothing against the chill. I poured the steaming rich brew into a blue NASA mug my son brought home from his visit to space camp; a second cup was poured for the officer who would presently come by to take me to the crime scene. My children then lined up against the frost-etched window, the younger kids squealing in delight at the flashing blue beacons, my eldest child more somber—he knows the implications of such nocturnal visits.

Like the commute home earlier, the ride to the crime scene was inordinately long. Upon my arrival at the scene, I was met by one of my favorite homicide detectives, who, instead of his usual smile, greeted me with a touch of ironic formality: "Evening, Dr Davis. Kind of you to come out on such a cold night." The freezing rain was coming down harder now as we stood beside the police cars; the faint smell of wood smoke wafting on the air from somewhere nearby reminded me of what

I was missing at home. The wipers of the police cars began to move ever more slowly as the windshields began to freeze. Of the dozen or so people at the scene, I noticed that only the uniformed officers and I were not shivering, as we were the only ones wearing hats, they with their standard issue, I in my trademark black Pendleton given to me years ago by Kathleen. It is an affectation that has earned me some gentle ribbing from colleagues, but tonight it stood me in good stead.

"Medical Examiner's here. Let 'im through!" barked one of the officers as I ducked beneath the yellow cordon tape. Glancing across the road, I noted the benumbed faces of individuals identified by the police as the murdered woman's daughter and son-in-law, their staring eyes caught in the blue strobe lights of the police cars.

Familiar questions peppered me as I crossed the threshold of the unheated ramshackle house of the woman lying dead on her living room floor. "How long has she been dead, Doc? What was used to hit her? Do you think she was killed here or moved from somewhere else?" As is my custom, I examined as much of the scene as I could before turning my attention to the body and attempting to answer the questions.

After breaking into her house, the assailant had beaten this 80-year-old woman over the head and strangled her. The detective and I meticulously went over her body, photographing and documenting any trace evidence that could possibly link a suspect to the crime. Dried blood spattered the floor and the wall adjacent to her head. The detective and I conversed quickly and quietly as we worked: we've shared many similar scenes before. Our breath condensed in the chill air like tiny clouds about our heads. We carefully avoided the overturned furniture and ransacked contents of the house as we continued our methodical work.

After two hours there was little else I could do to contribute to the investigation before the autopsy began, my major finding being the bloody print on the woman's chest of what appeared to be a man's sneaker. Now shivering, I beat a hasty retreat to the squad car. On the way home, the officer driving me and I discussed the particular brutality of this crime and the unnerving observation that, though they lived close by, this widow's daughter and son-in-law had not checked on her for weeks. She had in fact been dead for some time.

I arrived home just in time to help put the children to bed. Kathleen greeted me warmly, but since it had been a long week for her as well, she retired to our room and was soon fast asleep. I joined her in slumber only after listening to the rain still pelting the roof and ruminating on that lonely old woman, dead in her home for weeks before anyone noticed.

The next morning my partners performed the all-important autopsy. The postmortem examination had actually begun at the crime scene with the gathering of evidence such as the bloody shoe print; in fact, such a piece of evidence linking a possible murderer to the crime became the linchpin for the entire case. My partner and the pathology resident meticulously moved from the head to the toes of the victim, documenting all evidence of trauma and natural disease. The resident then startled me with a statement, echoing verbatim my thoughts of the night before, that she was upset by the thinness of the veneer of our civilization. She asked me with some distress, "When do you get to the point where such cases don't affect you?" My reply was one I have given on many occasions: "Although one has to remain totally dispassionate during the course of the autopsy in order to remain an objective observer and recorder, each one affects me to one extent or another." I paused and added, "One of the most important things you can do as a death investigator is to acknowledge the emotional toll that such cases take. Should they cease to take such a toll, you have to step back and assess your reasons for engaging in such a profession."

After the autopsy was done late that morning, I signed out to my partner and hopped into my car for the short trip to my synagogue. There on Saturday mornings, when I am not on duty, I partake in a weekly study of the Torah, the first five books of the Hebrew Bible, and of the Talmud, the texts of Jewish law assembled more than 12 centuries ago. Not just an intellectual challenge, it is a course of study that immerses me in the millennia of history. As I entered the study room filled with male and female students ranging in age from 16 to 90, I was greeted with the ancient Hebrew salutation of Shabbat Shalom: "A peaceful Sabbath to you."

I wish that it were so.

First Encounter

Daniel J. McCullough III

For almost a year of my life, death meant cadavers. Between gross anatomy, neuroanatomy, and microanatomy, I spent four of five weekday afternoons last year in a cool laboratory full of cadavers. Despite my initial apprehension, I grew more and more comfortable with the bodies until I truly felt that I knew Death: what it looked like, smelled like, felt like against the back of my hand. I *knew* Death.

Death is dead bodies. Their skin is waxy, their organs are a uniform gray, they smell like preservative. Death is dead. But I realize now that in all the time I spent dissecting cadavers, I was distanced from Death. I have since seen Death, and that is not what it looked like.

The night I saw Death started pleasantly enough. I was to join my father in Boston for dinner and a Celtics game. We decided to meet near the Boston Garden and walk to the North End for our dinner. The North End of Boston is the Italian section. Its winding streets lined by three-story brownstones are commonly known as the safest in New England. The area is a throwback to the city neighborhoods of yesteryear where everyone knows everyone else, where people live their whole lives on the same street on which they were born. There is a real sense of community living there and, for an "inner" section of a large city, a conspicuous lack of street violence. We found one of the many quiet family restaurants on Hanover Street and went in.

We had just about finished dinner when a young couple burst through the restaurant door and dove into a corner, the man covering the woman.

"Everybody down on the floor!" screamed the owner. "They're shooting in the streets!" My father slid off his chair and I joined him on the floor. This can't be happening, I thought. This is the North End. There must be some kind of mistake.

Several long minutes passed. Then someone outside started screaming about blood. The owner peeked out the window. My dad, an emergency medical technician, shouted, "Does someone out there need medical help?"

"Oh God yes!" a girl screamed back. "He's covered with blood!"

We stood and cautiously made our way to the door. Inching it open, we stepped out to the sidewalk. As the door closed behind us, I looked up, and I saw Death—alive—for the first time.

It was sitting on the chest of a young man of my age who was 10 feet away, slumped on the passenger seat of a car—its door open—at the curb. His head was tilted back as though he were resting. His desperate breathing was raspy. It seemed as if he were trying to speak, but with every effort, blood gushed from his mouth. A man—possibly a police officer—knelt next to him, pressing what looked like a sweatshirt against the young man's throat.

"He's finished," my dad said, shaking his head. "Poor kid."

"But he's alive!" The medical student in me protested. I *knew* he was alive. I knew he was young. And I knew all too well how resilient such a body was. I was the one who had studied it, taken it apart, admired its refined effectiveness. I knew that compression would minimize the bleeding until an ambulance arrived, that a transfusion would replace the lost blood. I knew that we were 20 blocks from one of the best hospitals in the world. There, physicians could easily arrest the probable hypovolemic shock. A few sutures, emergency surgery, surely he would make it. I knew it.

"He's gone," my dad said.

What did he know? I glared at him, then turned back to the young man. His chest heaved beneath the red wetness of his shirt. His stomach muscles contracted, then relaxed. He arched his back, coughed a bloody cough, then all was terribly still. More police arrived. The street began to fill with people while police tried to keep them away from the car. Sirens. Lights. An ambulance arrived, the crowd slowly moved aside, but my eyes never left the body.

"It happens fast," I mumbled.

"Yeah," my dad replied. "It's a fine line."

We turned and walked away, each absorbed in his own thoughts. Finally I stopped and said, "I think I just had my first look at the enemy. The one I'm training to fight the rest of my life."

"Death?" he asked.

"Yeah," I replied, and continued walking.

A few hours later we said our good-byes. Dad headed home, and I drove to school. A light drizzle had begun.

I stopped my car on top of a hill near school, got out, and stood looking out over the city, over the lights, over the buildings, looking over the living and the dead. I swore out loud at Death, and I cursed the violence in my country. I told Death that I knew it was going to win the war in the end but that I didn't care. I would be damned if I was going to let it win all the battles.

God Save the Child

Charles Atkins, MD

On *60 Minutes*, or maybe it was *Dateline* or *20/20*, I watched a story about research that had been done on the effects of parental deprivation. It was a sad feature with wide-eyed baby chimpanzees that clung to rag-doll "mothers" and hard-metal maternal scarecrows as various stressors were introduced into their cages by semisadistic researchers. In one, a chimp with no mother, or mother equivalent, lay huddled in the corner rocking and banging its head against the bars. The narrator drew inferences to early development in humans. He talked about orphans in Romania and failure to thrive. I thought about Connecticut and my daily evaluations.

"Tell me where you were born," I begin, with pen poised, knowing that if I want to keep the story straight I will have to write fast.

"Chicago/New York/L.A./a suburb outside Boston, but I was only there for a couple months."

"How come?"

"Well then my mother_____."

And I fill in the blank. "She died." "She left." "She got arrested." "She couldn't handle me so she gave me to my aunt/grandmother/a friend."

"And where was your dad?"

"He_____."

Fill in the blank. "I never knew him." "He left." "He got arrested." "They got divorced." "He did drugs." "He beat her." "He beat me." "He molested me."

"And then what?"

"We moved."

"To where?"

"To Chicago/New York/L.A./a suburb outside Boston, but we were only there for . . ."

And like chasing a rabbit through my backyard I dodge and move with the twists and the turns in the story. The child grows and reaches puberty.

"We were in New Jersey for a few years staying with my aunt, but then_____."

And another blank gets filled. "I got arrested." "I started doing drugs." "I was raped." "I reported my mother to DCF for hitting me." "I was put in a foster home." "I went to the shelter."

"How come?"

"I don't know."

"You have no idea?" I persist.

"Well, maybe_____."

And so it goes.

"Where do you want to be now?" I ask.

"Back with my mom/dad/aunt/grandmother."

"But I thought you said that he/she hit you/beat you/didn't respect you/raped you."

"But it could be different."

"What would it take?" I ask.

"Well, if he/she would stop taking drugs/hitting me/hitting her/ touching me/working so much/sleeping around so much it would be better."

"What else would you like?"

"To not be sad/to not cry all the time/to go back to school/to not do drugs/for my mom/dad to want me."

"How do you get there from here?"

"I don't know."

"Do you think that things will get better?"

"Yes/no/I don't know/maybe."

"Do you ever think about what you want to be when you're older?"

"An actor/a nurse/a teacher/a doctor/someone who looks after kids/a farmer."

I write it all down, taking hen-scratch notes. I'll dictate the whole thing later and try to keep the order straight: three or four years with both parents, then a separation and then the divorce, the first move, the second move, the stepfathers and the mother's boyfriends, the removal from the house, the first brush with the law, the first involvement with DCF, then the string of foster homes. I will track the sexual history, the first abuse, the first crush that progressed to intercourse at a precocious age, and the string of sexually transmitted diseases—some that can be treated and some that may be fatal. I will look at the child, in a child's body, and I will see a child. He/she will be neatly dressed and will talk freely about the abuse and the fissures that split the family further and further apart. He/she will smile and laugh and show a strange disconnection with the material they talk about. A few may start to cry, but by and large the stories come with little of that. If it weren't for the referral to a psychiatrist, I might never know how wrong things had gone. But I have read the referral form and so I head below the surface.

"You feel sad/angry/unhappy?" I will prod.

"Sometimes."

"You ever feel so bad that you wish you weren't alive?"

"Sometimes."

"How do you handle that?"

Soon, I am being shown limbs laced with scars from late-night episodes with razor blades and knives. I am told of psychiatric hospitalizations that followed overdose attempts, intentional car crashes, self-inflicted wounds, and threats of suicide. Many have come close to dying, some on more than one occasion.

"How long were you in the hospital?" I ask.

"Three days the first time, a week the second, maybe the same the third."

"Do you still think about killing yourself?"

"Sometimes."

"How often do you think about it?"

"Every day."

"What stops you?"

"I don't know."

"Do you see yourself ever feeling better?"

"Not really."

"That must be pretty discouraging."

"Tell me about it," he/she will say, while mustering a sad and knowing smile.

By the end of the interview we will have agreed on an initial course of treatment—of course, this will need to be cleared with his/her managed care company—but that's a different essay. The program that the child will enter for a few days or a few weeks will attempt to provide stability, guidance, role models, and techniques for handling anger and depression, and possibly medication. The treatment team will look at the child's goals and try to salvage any remnants of a family that might be viable. We will meet with the mother/father/aunt/grandmother/DCF worker/teacher/probation officer. We will try to teach parenting/frustration tolerance/forgiveness/boundary setting. In essence, we will attempt to construct a cloth mother out of whatever pieces of social attachment the child may have and that we might be able to create. We hold little illusion about the impact we can have in such a short time, but as the scientists and chimpanzees demonstrated, a cloth or hard-metal mother is better than no mother at all.

Frozen in Time

Robert Burns, MD

I should not be here. I feel guilty, out of place. Much like a teenager getting ready to buy liquor with a forged ID card, I look around the room and make sure I don't know anyone. The shop is busy, the customers look like me, my friends. Everyone else looks out of place too.

"I've got it. This is the one for you."

The owner places it on a velvet-lined tray and slides it toward me. I think about the merchants of Paris, refusing to exchange money with customers because it reduces the transaction to a business deal. This merchant is no different. I am no longer just a potential buyer. I am a friend. I am welcomed into the family. I hesitate just a second, then pick up the piece of hardened steel and hold it in my right hand. The Browning nine-millimeter is heavy, heavier than I thought. It is cold. I rub my fingers along the smooth barrel. I wrap both hands around the handle and draw it toward me, pointing the barrel toward the ceiling. The smell of the steel enters my nostrils, and a sudden rush of warmth penetrates my hands.

―――――――――

I do not want to be surprised. "What've ya got?" I ask as I walk down the hall and out the door of the emergency room. I pause. The cold night air enters my lungs, stings my nostrils, and revives me if only for a few minutes. It is Saturday night, and the ER is busier than usual. The checks are late this month, and people had to make a choice between food and medicines. It is my first break in eight hours and the next six already look worse. A few stars show through the clear sky. I take another breath, savoring its crisp freshness before dealing with the task at hand.

The paramedic has not answered my question. We have gone through this ritual before. Each of us has our refuge from the insanity of everyday work, of the world, and he knows mine. I will pay for these few moments of tranquillity when I enter the ambulance. He allows me my time, alone. Free. I walk toward the ambulance.

"Gunshot," he finally says, timing the words to the instant my foot touches the rear step of the ambulance. "Lovers' spat. Close range." There is no emotion in his voice.

He reaches in and turns on the light and I climb into the van. Medical supplies dangle from the cabinets and encroach into the already-too-small space. The overhead light flickers, plunging the cabin into intermittent darkness. A black body bag is strapped on the stretcher. I put down my paperwork. I hold onto the leather strap and pull the zipper.

The last remaining heat from the lifeless body escapes into the frigid March night. I open the bag, stretching a strand of thick, dark blood from the inside cover. The blood smells damp, metallic. I touch his neck, feeling for the pulse that his vacant eyes tell me has long since stopped. I usually check for five seconds, a perfunctory examination that matches the bureaucratic formality, not wanting it to last longer than necessary. Tonight, I search for the extinguished beat for 20, 30 seconds, staring into his still, brown eyes. His face appears pained. A crease across his brow, the muscles of his jaw tight, a grimace to his lips, frozen in time, at least until the mortician eases his suffering for eternity. He becomes my patient, and I want to know his history. What happened, or more importantly, why did it happen? What were his last thoughts? Did it hurt? Was his last vision of this life his lover at close range? I move my hand across his eyes and close them, trying to bring peace to us both.

"Remember, it's just the two of you. You never aim a gun unless your intention is to kill."

My instructor slaps my shoulder and steps aside, and I extend my arms above my head. The glasses are in place. The sweet, slightly acrid smell of gunpowder fills the air. Ear plugs are in place. I hear the melodic muted exploding of shells in the distance. I lower my arms. Elbows locked. The gun is level with my eyes. Twenty-five feet beyond the sight is a paper torso.

Concentric circles radiate from the chest, the heart, an imaginary vortex ready to pull the missiles to their target.

He was wrong. There is no other rational explanation for it. He was at the wrong place at the wrong time. I had been with him minutes earlier. It was his turn to drive to the hockey game, and he had left me in my driveway. He flashed his headlights at me as I entered the house, and his car disappeared into the cloud of exhaust left in the cold winter night as the tires crunched the gravel. I remember when I was a child that sound gave me comfort. It meant my father was finally home. We were all home. Safe.

He was wrong. Why did he stop for money on the way home? It could have waited until morning. The bank of floodlights, in place for safety, illuminated his every step. As if he were an actor on stage, his audience watched from the shadows as he filled his wallet with the money and moved to his car. And then they followed him home.

He was wrong. He should have left his porch light on when he left the house. It would have protected him. When he pulled into his driveway he would have been home. Safe.

He was wrong. All he had to do was hand them the wallet. It was probably all they wanted. Give them what they want, the police always say. It was just paper, plastic, and leather. Nothing more. No heirlooms. No memories. Disposable, like a life. He must have punched and struggled with them. It is the only rational explanation. Why else was he pushed to the ground, the barrel of the handgun placed at his temple, and the trigger pulled?

I grip the handle. The muscles in my arms tense. My finger pulls against the trigger, but stops.

"Squeeze the trigger," he says.

Sweat drips into my eyes. The target, just paper, plastic, and metal, blurs beyond my sight. Squeeze the trigger. My finger cramps. I feel the blood pulse in my fingers. I close my eyes. The rhythmic beating of my heart increases, my pulse pounds in my neck, in my temples, and finally in my skull. I see the torso. My palms sweat and I loosen my grip. I open my eyes, the torso is closer. It's moving, no longer just a target but a body, rushing toward me to challenge. My arms tense; I grip the pistol, lowering the site to the center of the chest. I pull the trigger and a deafening shot explodes. The gun pushes back against me; I step back to maintain my balance. A curl of smoke escapes from the barrel as shredded paper gently floats to the ground. The target sways from its hanger, a hole ripped through the center.

My arms drop to my sides; the gun feels heavier. My pulse slows; I wipe the sweat from my eyes. A chill rushes through my body, and I need to vomit.

"Again," the instructor says. "Do it again. The second one is always easier."

Thanks for the Memories

Perhaps the most common type of manuscript that I receive falls into the category I call "my favorite patient." (Actually, some could be classified "my most difficult patient," but both have one thing in common: patients made an impact and changed lives.) There is the child with arthritis who gives his rheumatologist an impromptu backrub ("Friday Afternoon"); the migrant farm worker with malignant hypertension whose frustrated physician is unable to effectively treat her because of the woman's transient status ("Until the Peppers"); the shy and troubled young man with severe psoriasis whose treatment plan includes not only effective medications but compassion ("Flaky"); and the young girl with full-blown AIDS, whose courage, humor, and dignity motivate her caregivers to use everything in their power to save her, to no avail ("The Little Picture"). In "The Captain," a retired sea captain agrees to undergo treatment and hospitalization after a heart attack only after he is convinced his physician was a member of his crew on a Victory ship during the 1950s. These few essays represent only a small fraction of the millions of patient-physician encounters that take place every day, each as unique as the individual players themselves.

R.K.Y.

Friday Afternoon

John T. Lynn III, MD

It had been a long week—by anyone's definition. My wife and I had recently separated after 17 years of marriage. I had moved into an efficiency apartment, less than a tenth the size of my house, where I was learning, slowly, to entertain my two children.

The last person on my schedule that week was a new patient named Walter Johnson. I took his chart from the nurse and called for "Mr Johnson." In the waiting room, a woman gave her little boy a bewildered look.

"This is Walter," the woman said, pointing to her son.

"I'm Dr Lynn. Happy to meet you. I guess I was expecting an older gentleman," I explained as I shook the boy's hand. I led mother and son to the examining room, where Walter began to climb on and off the examination table as if it were a jungle gym. The paper on the table crinkled with each of his movements.

"Calm down, Walter," his mother said, then turned to me. "Doctors make him nervous."

"Me too," I replied. "Walter, how old are you? I'll bet you're 10 or 11."

He smiled and waved five fingers at me. Young children always love to be mistaken for older, a fact I take advantage of to build rapport with them.

Walter continued to explore the room. He pulled the blood pressure cuff off the wall, then inspected the stack of fresh gowns in the cabinet.

"Walter looks pretty vigorous to me," I observed. "What's he doing in an arthritis specialist's office?"

His mother explained that Walter had been having knee pain for two years, worse in the mornings and at bedtime, and she'd noticed some swelling and warmth in both knees recently. He didn't have any other symptoms, and ibuprofen seemed to relieve his discomfort.

Watching Walter navigate the room was enough of an examination for me, but I did, probably for his mother's benefit, coax him onto the table. All of his joints moved well without tenderness, and his knees, if anything, were a little ticklish.

I explained to his mother that Walter probably had a mild case of pauciarticular juvenile rheumatoid arthritis and that his pain and swelling would gradually improve without any lasting damage to the joints. I recommended that he take ibuprofen daily. I considered teaching him special exercises for his knees, but this kid did not need more exercise. I finished, asking his mother to have an ophthalmologist examine Walter's eyes for the subtle inflammation that can occur in a small number of children with this condition.

"Can I have my husband in to hear this too?" the mother asked.

"Sure," I replied through tightly smiling lips. Being asked to repeat my discussion was a little like approaching the finish line at the end of the mile run and being told by the coach to sprint another lap. I sent Walter to bring back his father from the waiting room.

I told the whole family about juvenile rheumatoid arthritis, and I described how the tests done by their family physician helped to rule out other possible causes of Walter's arthritis. Midway through the discussion, I felt two little hands rubbing my tight shoulder girdle and upper back. I wasn't sure whether I should accept a massage from a patient, but it felt good, so I continued talking.

His parents smiled, then laughed.

"I've never seen Walter take to anybody like this," his mother declared. "He never scratches our backs."

Hearing his name, Walter became self-conscious and began to pace the room again. I told his father that his son's knees would gradually improve, and I rose from my stool.

"When do you want to see Walter again?" his father asked.

"Every Friday afternoon would be great. But an appointment in six months will be just fine."

Leek Soup

James F. Gardner III, MD

Cecille first walked into my office dressed in blue stretch pants and a flowered blouse under a full-length camel's hair coat. Her graying, soft brown hair was cut Dutch-boy style. Everything about her suggested middle America except for a mink coif she wore regally.

"I never expected to live this long," she said, after exchanging initial pleasantries.

I was caught off-guard by her remark and laughed nervously for lack of any comeback. Her daughter, who had accompanied Cecille into the examination room, rolled her eyes as one does who has heard something countless times before.

"Now, Mother. God's not ready for you yet," came the practiced reply.

Cecille was born in 1900. She doesn't look a day over 65. Her slender records reveal only two medical problems: hypertension and hyperlipidemia. Her blood pressure is easily controlled with an ACE inhibitor, but her total cholesterol has never dipped below 300 mg/dL. Previous physicians fussed at her about this. Over the years her understanding of the involved physiology took a sharp turn: she is now sure that butter and eggs make her blood pressure rise.

Her cholesterol values concerned me at first. They needn't have. All of her elder relatives lived to be at least octogenarians. And they did it on a diet anathematized by modern medicine. Cecille loves good food, rich food, haute cuisine. She was, you see, born in Belgium.

She is fluent in French, of course, but speaks English without a trace of accent. With each passing visit, she and I talk more of food and wine, and less of calories and atherogenesis. She regales me with recipes for sauces to die for. I asked if there were any local French restaurants she approved of. She said she rarely eats out, preferring to cook for herself.

"The Belgian way is so much tastier than the French," she sniffed.

It was during one such medicoculinary encounter that Cecille discussed leek soup. It sounded so easy that I wrote the ingredients on a prescription pad. I tried to pin her down on proportions and procedures but without much success. Like all great chefs, I thought, she cooks by feel. Very well. How hard could it be?

A leek is a strange vegetable. It looks like a chive with a glandular problem. It is surprisingly dirty. Nevertheless, I was committed. Into fresh, bubbling chicken stock went coarsely chopped potato, onion, and leek. Pinches of salt and pepper, and a bay leaf, followed. A suitable simmer later, all contents (minus the bay leaf) were transferred to a food processor—Cecille's wink to modern convenience that I found shocking. A flip of a switch turned my work into a roiling suspension that I hoped would become gourmet greatness. What emerged was a thin, green, Amazonian ooze. Not unpleasant to taste, but certainly a textural failure. Out of embarrassment I never told Cecille of my attempt to cop her soup. In retrospect, I believe less broth, more potato, and a lower setting on the Osterizer® could yet yield the bisque I yearn for.

Cecille was born in Liège, a large town near Belgium's border with Germany. Her family had been well-to-do until, on what seemed a lark, her father sold all of their ancestral lands and uprooted the family to Alberta, Canada. They drifted for years until Cecille's father decided his blossoming daughter should benefit from a more polished education. She and a brother were shipped off to Europe, arriving in Belgium in 1914. Five months later, the Huns smashed through the Low Countries during the initial salvos of World War I.

Cecille spent the entire war with her grandparents under German occupation. She recalls how she took barge rides into a nearby hamlet to visit her country cousins. On each return trip, they would sew cheeses and sausages into the lining of her ratty-looking coat.

"I was such a skinny rail of a girl, the German guards never gave me a second look," she said. In this manner her family fared much better than most of their city-dwelling neighbors.

She remembers the times her family huddled in the cellar while German troops made sweeps of the neighborhood looking for food or contraband. It was generally known that if you stayed out of sight, the soldiers left you alone. For some reason on such a day, Cecille's grandfather insisted on preparing tea upstairs. Hiding below, the family heard two gunshots. Fears for his safety mounted when, several minutes later, the shriek of the tea-kettle went unanswered. He had been shot—through the open kitchen window. Contents of the home went untouched. Cecille tells this story in a terse, emotionless style, belied by a single tear in her medial canthus. Seventy-five years have not dimmed a granddaughter's love.

Happier times found Cecille living the life of an artist and schoolteacher in Hawaii. She recalls the Sunday morning she started an early breakfast for her children. She stepped outside to pick up the newspaper and heard a deep drone to the northwest. The noise belonged to chevrons of low-flying Japanese planes that proceeded to pass over her cottage.

"I knew right away they weren't ours," she said. "I could see rising suns everywhere. Some of the pilots actually waved at me, so close they were!" Minutes later she heard distant concussions coming from the harbor at Pearl.

I relish my visits with Cecille. Each one a chance to tap living, breathing history. What a survivor. This soul whose passage on earth reaches through the two greatest human cataclysms of the 20th century. A tragic heroine in the classical mold. Carried by unyielding currents and tossed about by forces beyond control. Yet, not rudderless. Between the upheavals, she too has known marriage, childbirth, divorce, bereavement. We can all relate to such a life. A common hand on the tiller.

I long ago stopped worrying about Cecille's cholesterol. To a life force such as hers, a chylomicron is a gnat. Each time she leaves my office, the nurses laugh as she snaps off her best line.

"I never expected to live this long, you know."

"Nor so well," I whisper.

The History of Crete

Selma Harrison Calmes, MD

It was a horrible day when I learned about the history of Crete. It was Friday, the beginning of a holiday weekend. I was the anesthesiologist on-call and faced four straight days of work. The week had already brought an overwhelming number of trauma cases to our county hospital, and the upcoming weekend would only bring more. All week I'd lived in my scrubs, consuming my customary tuna fish sandwiches while on the run to the ICU or ED to pick up a critically ill patient. Paperwork was piled to staggering heights in my office. Personal financial worries added to my feeling of going under.

It was about 6 PM before we finally got to Mr Nicklaus, who was to have a cysto. He was 51 years old and a physical wreck. He had cancer of the larynx, severe bronchiectasis, and Rendu-Osler-Weber syndrome. He'd arrived five days before from a small hospital in the nearby southern Sierra community where he lived. He'd checked into that hospital, pulled a handgun out of his suitcase, and shot himself in the head five times. He blew out an eye, but miraculously he had survived. We repaired his orbit wound.

I first saw him as he lay on the cysto table. He was a tiny, shriveled-up man covered with the purple spots of the Rendu-Osler-Weber syndrome. His long white hair was in utter disarray, and he was amazingly cantankerous. He complained loudly about the "cretins" who were taking care of him, about the pain in his orbit, about his sore neck, about being cold, about his painful bedsores. He was precisely the sort of patient I couldn't face then, one I'd like to put to sleep just to keep him quiet. But because of his scheduled operation, his health problems, and the facial defect from his orbital wound, a spinal was in order.

He continued to complain as we sat him up for the spinal. His ten-inch-long laminectomy scar greeted me, adding to our problems and annoying me further. Fortunately, I got the spinal in quickly. I had trouble hearing his heart and breath sounds while trying to place a precordial stethoscope. I told him, with a touch of bitterness (owing to the state of my life), that I couldn't hear his heart and was sure he'd lost it. Surprisingly he joked back, "In Avalon," the resort island off the California coast and the subject of the World War II–era popular song. That was the first clue that Mr Nicklaus might be more than he appeared.

The surgeon was ready, and I gave Mr Nicklaus some intravenous narcotic for sedation. He said he felt warm for the first time and soon stopped complaining. He told me he'd been stationed on Avalon during World War II and had flown P-38s off the West Coast, searching for enemy invaders. He criticized various military strategies used during the war, and declared he had had five wives. As a merchant marine he had traveled extensively, he said, and then opined his choice of the five best cities in the world. At last he fell asleep, and I had a little peace.

Suddenly he woke and bellowed, "Have you ever studied the history of Crete?" "Not recently," I replied, inwardly groaning that I didn't have time for *anything* now, much less studying an ancient civilization. A lecture on Crete's cultural and artistic achievements promptly followed. Mr Nicklaus' travels had led him there, a jewel in "the wine-dark sea," as he informed me Homer had written in the *Odyssey*. The remains of this 3000-year-old society enthralled Mr Nicklaus. Most exciting was the Palace at Knossos, capital of the empire established by King Minos, son of Zeus. He described the palace's lavatories, complete with a flushing apparatus, modern-style bath-tubs, and a water supply system made of baked clay pipes. He talked of the fine artwork he'd seen, vases of soapstone with carved sea creatures and the marvelous painted walls. He told me of the palace's excavation in 1900. He was simply crazy about ancient Crete.

We talked through the whole operation. When it ended, he announced he was starving for cornflakes and ice cream, which the resident then ordered. I finally went home—to a bowl of cornflakes instead of my tuna sandwich—wiser about the history of Crete and not quite so irritable.

That wasn't the end of Mr Nicklaus and me. He returned to the OR several days later for a prostate resection, demanding me for his anesthesiologist. And once again this amazing-looking man poured out fascinating stories of his life, argued his views on world events, and asked for cornflakes and ice cream.

I saw Mr Nicklaus several times after his surgery, my interest piqued by the contrast between his physical appearance and what was inside his mind. He sent messages asking me to visit, and I did when I could. During one such visit, he said he'd had a dream about the two of us. We'd been working a jigsaw puzzle together, not competitively but cooperatively, and what a wonderful feeling that had given him. Could he, I wondered, be deciding to put the pieces of *his* life together? And if so, was I helping him to do this? I hoped so. His grooming improved, he started to put on some weight, and eventually he was discharged to a nursing home in town.

He wrote me soon after his discharge, complaining about his caretakers and the food and pleading that I visit. At that time I had to leave town but sent him a note that I'd see him when I got back. It was several days after my return before I was able to call the nursing home. I was shocked to learn he had died.

I searched the newspapers, from the days I'd been away, for an obituary about this man and his extraordinary life. But there was nothing: no obituary, nothing to mark his life or his death. He seemed simply to have vanished.

I've done a lot of thinking about Mr Nicklaus. He probably hadn't really wanted to die when he shot himself. After all, he had checked into a hospital in the first place, where he would be found and treated promptly. I happened along and made contact with him, and somehow I think he recovered some will to live. I suspect he may then have lost that will in the nursing home. Did the nursing home have cornflakes and ice cream on demand? Such small pleasures seemed extremely important to him. I wonder now if my letter—delaying my visit—had been a factor in his death.

My letter from Mr Nicklaus is in a drawer with other treasured items from my life, a small reminder of that ruined body that still had marvelous things inside. And it reminds me of me at that time: when I was so discouraged, Mr Nicklaus took me to another world for a while. I now view difficult patients in a new and different way; I wonder what their past lives might have been, what they might be able to teach me.

I've read several books on the history of Crete; Mr Nicklaus was right. Ancient Crete was quite amazing. When I wander museums, I find myself drawn to those antiquities, and I remember this man and his love of this ancient civilization. I'll never forget Mr Nicklaus and the history of Crete, especially when I'm eating a bowl of cornflakes.

House Calls

Ronald F. Galloway, MD

The first time I saw him, Mr Henry was standing in front of a mirror, his back to the door of his hospital room, tinkering with his electric razor and fixing to shave. I called his name; he turned, put down his razor, smiled, and reached out to grasp my hand. He was tall, skinny as a rail, a bit stoop-shouldered, but he moved about pretty spryly.

As a thoracic surgeon, I had been asked to see Mr Henry regarding a possible resection for a lemon-sized tumor in his left lung. He was 80 years old at the time. I had already seen his chest film and reviewed his chart and was, I admit, trying to think of a gentle way to explain to him that, at his age, he would not likely do well after major chest surgery. My preconceived notion was reinforced by the fact that he had been admitted with a proved diagnosis of carcinoma of the prostate. However, his smile and his firm handshake cut through that preconception, so I explained to him all the ifs, ands, and buts of a pulmonary lobectomy and informed him that his attending urologist planned a total orchiectomy at the same sitting. At the end of my detailed talk I paused and asked for questions. He had only one: "When do we do this?" I told him. He smiled again and said, "I'm ready."

Mr Henry tolerated both surgical procedures well, had no complications, and soon went home. At his follow-up visit at my office a few weeks later, I learned that his wife's health was poor, that he didn't drive a car especially well, and that his coming to my office for checkups was difficult at best. So, I told him that on occasion I drive to the South Carolina coast and that his town was on the way. I offered to stop by to visit him from time to time. He seemed surprised but obviously appreciative that I would volunteer to do this.

Some weeks later I drove through that small town, followed his directions to its outskirts, and found the house trailer on concrete blocks that

Mr and Mrs Henry called home. The yard was well kept—a small, neat garden decorated one corner. I hadn't called for an "appointment" but had presumed that his wife's poor health kept Mr Henry close to home. I knocked on the door and was greeted by Mr Henry with a smile as big as all outdoors and his special warm handshake. I examined him, noted that he was doing quite well, and spent a while just visiting with them both. As I left, I felt absolutely wonderful.

I've returned to the Henrys several times since that first encounter. They seem to enjoy my visits, and each trip has been an unqualified blessing for me.

It has occurred to me that I could, if I wished, file a claim with Medicare for reimbursement for these 72-mile (144 miles round-trip) "house calls." But, the thought of the hassle the Medicare people would give me and the probability that they wouldn't believe I made 72-mile house calls in the first place have deterred me. Then, too, the frozen boiled peanuts Mr Henry gave me on one trip, the tomatoes he promised me this summer, the pride he takes in showing me his garden, the look in his eyes when I appear at his door, and my personal "hands-on" knowledge that he continues to do well are worth far more than any amount I might be able to argue out of Medicare.

And there's no deductible to meet.

Another Language

Marcia Goldoft, MD

I don't suppose you speak Russian."

"Speak *Russian*? No." As an intern I'd learned that the city hospital's emergency room generated its share of unusual events, but this question sounded particularly strange. "Why?"

"There's a probable CHF here to admit," replied the ER intern. "Lungs a little wet, peripheral edema, the works. But she speaks what we believe is Russian. There's no one with her."

"Terrific." It was going to be one more impossible chore in the long night of admitting duty. "If she's stable enough for the ward, send her up."

Her chart was limited to an ER note and lab slips. A neighbor had called an ambulance but could inform the EMTs only that the elderly woman had knocked on his door and seemed to be having trouble breathing. He thought she had recently arrived from Russia and was living with a relative who frequently went out of town.

"Does anyone here speak Russian?" I asked at the nursing station, more out of an attempt at thoroughness than anticipating an affirmative answer. There was the expected shaking of heads. During the day the hospital had translators available on call for its many European patients, but at night we usually relied on family members for assistance.

Feeling aggravated at the additional difficulty in the middle of a busy evening, I walked to my new patient's hospital room. Sitting up in bed, in a hospital gown much too big for her, was a white-haired, frail, and apparently frightened woman. An IV was taped to one hand, and in the other she clutched a battered black purse.

"Hello," I smiled, hoping to reassure her. She said nothing, only continued to breathe with effort. We looked at each other for a moment, lacking any other means of communication. "Doctor," I said, pointing to myself. She nodded without losing her anxious expression. With gestures I showed her the stethoscope and indicated that I wanted to listen to her chest. Again she nodded.

The examination findings were consistent with mild congestive heart failure, as was the chest film. Even if we didn't know anything about her, we could still treat her medical problems. Standing at the nursing station, I wrote orders and started what would be an embarrassingly brief admission note.

"Excuse me, I heard you talking before. Do you need someone who speaks Russian?" A man had approached the counter where I was working. "I'm waiting for my wife, who's visiting her mother here, and overheard your problem."

"Do you speak Russian?"

He didn't but explained that he did speak some Yiddish and his father-in-law, who had accompanied him, knew Yiddish and Russian, although little English. Perhaps together they could manage to translate for me. As the patient watched I pulled some extra chairs into the room and beckoned the men in. The older man began talking, and after listening for a few minutes the patient started to speak. They spelled her name for me, and then I began the interview.

It was an abbreviated medical history, the questions going from me to the man to his father-in-law to the patient, the answers returning by the reverse path, her words coming slowly between strained breaths. I requested only the basic information about her heart, her lungs, her medications. English to Yiddish to Russian to Yiddish to English, and I could only hope that the shifts from language to language did not fragment the meanings between us.

"Has this happened before?" I asked. The woman had been hospitalized once in Kiev. Sometimes she had trouble breathing at night, particularly when her feet swelled.

I tried to determine what had worsened her symptoms. Prescribed medication had helped her breathe, but she had run out of pills that week. "The doctor told her to eat less salt," the younger man translated, "but she says that with canned food she doesn't know how much salt there is."

The woman opened her purse and took out a thin wallet. From it she carefully removed a photograph and a business card. I looked at the picture of a middle-aged man. "Who is this?"

"Her cousin," came the answer. "Her cousin on her mother's side." He was doing very well in this country, I learned, and had offered the woman refuge when things became so disturbed in Russia. If he hadn't been traveling on business that week, he would have gotten fresh food and the pills for her as he usually did.

There was a telephone number on his card. "Please tell her we'll call his office in the morning and get in touch with him."

I imposed on my translators for just a few more minutes. "Could you please explain that this is an IV line to give her medicine like the pills? The green tube carries oxygen to help her breathe better." Surely they did not know the right translation for some of the words, even when I gave them the simplest possible descriptions, but she seemed to understand, and her eyes became less troubled. Thanking the men for their help, I added a more complete admission note to her chart and went on to other duties.

Her voice seemed to follow me, the accent and rhythm and inflections bringing thoughts of my own grandmother. She too had come to this country without knowledge of English and had never spoken it fluently. There were many things I wanted to know, thinking of these two women who had fled to the uncertainty of an unknown country rather than remain in their homelands. I wanted to understand what they had left and how they had found the courage to do so, how it felt to be in a country where not even the language was anything familiar.

Later that night I walked through the darkened hospital corridors and stopped at my patient's room to see if she was responding to the diuretics. The woman was still awake but breathing much more easily, and as I listened through the stethoscope I knew her lungs were clearing. Afterward, in the dim light of the hospital room, she looked up at me. The wrinkles around her eyes deepened as she smiled for the first time. Reaching out, I took her veined hand and gently pressed her fingers, speaking to her in another language.

My Heroes

Nina K. Regevik, MD

I am frequently asked by friends and colleagues, "How do you manage to take care of patients with AIDS? How do you *do* it?" My ready answer has always been that, in spite of the horror of the illness, I have seen people behave like heroes. AIDS has robbed hundreds of thousands of the prime years of their too-short lives, but, like many tragedies, it has also revealed the true mettle of many, many wonderful people. As a physician working exclusively with HIV-related disease, I am continually amazed and at once humbled at the acts of courage and of humanity that surface daily during clinic and rounds. And many of these acts come from those I would least expect, a fact that reminds me of my own sometimes narrow perceptions and expectations.

Stephanie was no different from most of my patients, except that perhaps she suffered more. She experienced the vast array of conditions commonly seen in AIDS, and then some: disseminated *Mycobacterium avium-intracellulare, Pneumocystis carinii* pneumonia with recurrent pneumothoraces that required chest tubes, severe herpetic and fungal oropharyngeal-esophageal infections, wasting and unremitting diarrhea—her blood cultures revealed organisms that defied identification. Not unexpectedly, all of this was coupled with the anxious depression that we see in so many people who struggle with catastrophic illness. Nevertheless, she continued, with the love and encouragement of her family, to maintain her head-of-the-household position. She surprised our entire medical team with amazing resilience and survived years longer than even our most optimistic predictions.

Her final hospitalization proved to be a steady downhill course: severe pneumonia with ventilatory failure, complicated by the drugs, complicated by the complications, and on, and on, and on. Tacit acknowledgment grew between our team and her family that this, in fact, was Stephanie's last battle.

She was not to have an easy death. Seizures, thrombi, tumors, infections, liver and respiratory failure all would appear before the end. Two things did not change, however: her heart remained strong and regular, and her consciousness remained inexorably intact.

Bravely tolerating the tubes and the machines, she nodded vigorously when we asked if she was okay, should we do more tests, should we try new treatments. Stephanie wanted to survive, and only her courage—and that of her mother and children—gave us the resolve to continue with what must have caused her unimaginable pain and suffering, and only a small glimmer of hope. She wanted her best shot at life and we gave her that.

But for me the hardest thing to watch was Stephanie's 10-year-old son. He came to see her as much as he could, but his last visit, a few days before she died, will stay with me for many years. He arrived after school, laden backpack slung over one shoulder, to see his mother for what I'm sure he realized would be the last time. This little person received his mother's last touch from hands swollen and deformed by gangrene, her neck rigid from intractable meningitis, her lips caked and cracked with sores and cuts. How could he ever handle it? I wondered. But handle it he did. He stood by her bedside and told his mommy how much he loved her, over and over, keeping back his tears. He even managed to hug and kiss her—not so easy when mommy has tubes coming from her mouth and nose, tubes that are attached to big, scary machines.

Several days later I met him again, this time at his mother's funeral. My heart ached when I saw his brand-new suit and dress shoes, and his neatly combed hair, with a just slightly crooked part, betraying the fact that 10-year-old boys don't do so well when a mom isn't around.

His behavior was impeccable. He sat ramrod straight in the pew, barely moving, lips pressed together, eyes ahead. At the end of the service, the usual procession started: the casket carried slowly down the aisle with the family trailing just behind. During the few moments' pause as preparations were made to leave, there was not a sound in the huge church, save for a few muffled sobs. Suddenly, I heard the clatter of shoes on the marble floor. I looked up to see him running toward me. He threw his arms around my neck, and, as we locked in a hug, I heard his quavering, loud voice: "Thank you, Dr Nina, for taking care of my mommy."

All at once, it was quite clear how I "do it" every day and—most certainly—why.

Retrieval

Robert H. Lokey, MD

The small, narrow, walnut-paneled room had been used for routine ECGs before I joined the group. It was now transformed with pride (and much help from my wife) into a comfortable setting that bespoke, in my view, dignity and professional competence. Since it was still my very first week in the practice, I was not overly busy and I spent time looking about the place with satisfaction, trying to imagine how impressive it would seem to patients coming into it for the first time. Would they feel reassured (despite my newness)? Would they be intimidated by the few fine pieces Louise had provided for me (by self-denial and secret saving), like the small drop-leaf table, the leather chair?

I played out in my mind just how I would exercise the skills I had arduously acquired to put the patient at ease, then probe his or her concerns by interview and examination and, after reasoning through the data, confirm my analysis by the judicious use of laboratory investigation my residency had taught me. And then, voilà! A satisfied and relieved patient would go forth extolling my virtues and singing my praises. Bring them on. I was ready!

Inez walked in without an appointment and no previous record with us. Her insistence had overridden the receptionist's will, and I agreed to see her (after all, I had the time). She marched into my office, pulled the leather chair around to face me, and put both elbows on my desk. (In the back of my mind I realized she hadn't noticed the room's decor at all.) She looked me square in the eye and said, "All I want to know from *you* is this: Do I *have* to die?"

Her blunt and angry question took me aback. In the rehearsals I'd mentally indulged in earlier, *this* scene had not played. I scrutinized her closely before I attempted a response—she was intensely jaundiced, her skin was replete with spider angiomas, a fine tremor of the hands was apparent. An alcoholic! What ironic bad luck, I silently cursed. Of all the problems our species was prey to, chronic alcohol addiction was one I felt least sympathetic toward. My only sibling had succumbed to it, and his disintegration and demise had biased me, probably irrevocably, against anyone so afflicted ever being salvaged. My residency had done nothing to amend this view. What do I *do* with this situation?

I began with a vague statement about the inevitability of death for us all—but she impatiently interrupted: "I'm not talking about that stuff. I mean *now, soon!*" As I stumbled on, through the litany of the history taking, it rapidly evolved that she had already visited another local physician, who had told her that her drinking had doomed her and she might as well go home and keep drinking. Alarm had caused her to seek another opinion. It further came out that she was the main provider for her granddaughter, and the thought of having to leave the child in the care of someone else was devastating.

This woman's anguish touched me deeply and highlighted the discomfiture I was already feeling. From previous dealings with alcoholics at this stage, I felt the earlier judgment given her was true but likely to be slowly drawn out with hell-to-pay along the way. Yet, I felt strongly moved to offer her some kind of help. The physical examination confirmed the extent of suspected liver disease.

"I must tell you there is evidence of considerable liver damage," I said to her as gently as I could make that honest conviction sound.

"Do you mean I can't get better?" she asked.

"I mean it will require an enormous effort on your part. It will not be easy, and the main hope of recovery will rest chiefly with your determination." Even as I said these things my previous experiences made me feel her chance for improvement was dim.

"Let's get at it," she replied without hesitation.

She was admitted to the hospital for careful monitoring, as the customary program for withdrawal was initiated. Within hours she became increasingly agitated and uncooperative. During the first 24 hours she experienced some hallucinatory moments. Medication had to be given intravenously and restraints applied. During this worst time Inez fought her bonds, snarled epithets at everyone attending her, and glared unrecognizingly at me, as she showered me with curses and threats.

After this stormy time passed, and she leveled off clinically, we began to build a bridge of trust between us and she shared other dimensions of her life: a childhood of abuse and neglect. Frequent times, as an older child, she would take her younger sister in tow and find shelter in sheds and buildings for a night or two to escape the drunken rowdiness at home. She eventually resorted to alcohol herself, as a teenager. She had married a bootlegger (a revelation that did nothing for my optimism for her sustained recovery). After the accidental death of her daughter, Inez had assumed the care of her daughter's daughter. Her accounts also gave evidence that she possessed a belligerent toughness that might prove helpful, if properly directed. After a few days we discharged her and arranged for the necessary follow-ups. In those days there were not available the community-wide rehabilitation resources we have today.

Inez never touched alcohol again. By dogged pursuit of her reclamation of self, motivated by a need to give that self for the well-being of another, Inez steadily improved. Before a year had passed, her liver functions were normal and remained so; her granddaughter thrived in the loving attention provided, finished college, and continued her own journey with an example of strength and devotion as additional reservoirs to call upon, when needed.

And Inez? She died 27 years after our first meeting, of progressive coronary heart disease. The end was like the beginning—tough and determined with no self-pity.

And me? I was taught an invaluable lesson by this remarkable woman: that well-established scientific realities are certainly applicable to groups of people with shared conditions, but may fail to account for the possibilities within an individual human spirit. Inez showed me the power of sustained pursuit of the impossible.

The Captain

Seigfried J. Kra, MD

A few years ago, I received a telephone call from a patient of mine who seemed to be at her wits' end.

"My father is having chest pain. I know he's having a heart attack. He refuses to go to the hospital. What can I do?"

"If he refuses that is his own choice," I replied, "but let me talk to him."

A gruff voice came over the line. "You aren't going to convince me, Doctor, so don't waste your time. Just go to your golf game."

I ignored the last remark. "I don't want to convince you, Mr Ripchen. Just out of curiosity, what do you do, what kind of work?"

"What do I do? Doctor, I am a port captain . . . if you know what that means."

"Captain, I know what a port captain is. I was at sea." He remained silent so I continued. "I was a merchant seaman, Captain, a long time ago."

"Is that so?" he retorted.

"Yes. Have you ever heard of the *Mankato Victory?*"

"The *Mankato!*" he shouted. "That was my ship! My daughter put you up to this. Well, it won't work. I'm not going to the hospital, and I'm not going to your office!"

"Well, Captain Ripchen, I was on the *Mankato* and you will have to come here to find out what I did on that Victory ship."

To this day I don't know why I asked the man if he had ever heard of the *Mankato Victory*. It was so long ago that I worked for Marine State, a shipping company that carried cargo to Iceland, Wales, and Hamburg, Germany, on those old World War II Victory and Liberty ships.

"Listen, Buster, I *will* come to your office," he said, "but you'd better be telling the truth. Before I leave, tell me, what was the name of the radio operator on the *Mankato?*"

"'Sparky' was his name."

"We called *all* of them 'Sparky,'" he growled. "What did he look like?"

"Sparky? Well, he had red hair and a glass eye, and he was from Finland."

"Well, I'll be damned!" he yelled. "Sparky had red hair and a glass eye. What year were you on the *Mankato*?"

"1953 to 1954," I answered.

"Where did you ship out from?" he asked.

"The old Brooklyn Navy yard. Because of security reasons, we could come aboard only by taking a Moran tugboat. We had to climb a Jacob's ladder to get aboard. The Brooklyn was an important navy-operated ship-yard where the ships left with tanks and vehicles."

"That's correct, too. What were you, a security agent?" he asked.

"I'm not going to tell you unless you get someone to examine you," I insisted. "Captain, are you still having chest pain?"

"Not anymore. I feel fine."

"Listen, Captain, go to your local hospital. You don't need to come here."

"You're not going to convince me to go to a hospital. Now if you were on the *Mankato* in 1953," he continued, "tell me where we were that November."

"In the North Sea," I told him, "off Iceland in a horrendous storm. The ship nearly split in half, and we lost some cargo."

"My daughter put you up to this. She must have given you all of these details."

"No, sir. As a matter of fact, one of the men was so badly injured we had to change our course for Greenland," I said. "He was your first engineer, Robert something."

"Robert McCormick," he put in. "I'm coming right over. I have to see you, but don't think you're going to put me in the hospital."

It had been 30 years since I last saw him. He was as tall as I remembered, and as imposing. He wore a cap you could buy only in Bremerhaven, Germany, decorated with little pins representing all the ports he had visited. He obviously did not recognize me as he circled around, eyeing me up and down. He looked the same except his face was wrinkled, and his hair was gray. Then and now he reminded me of the late actor Raymond Massey.

After his third turn he suddenly slipped to the floor. I knelt to examine him. His heart was racing, and his blood pressure was at shock level. I called for an ambulance.

"I'm okay, Doc," he whispered, "just a little weak. I guess I will go to your hospital for a few days." He paused. "But only you can take care of me."

Despite my years of medical practice and involvement in the care of hundreds of persons with myocardial infarctions, waiting for an ambulance as I hover over a patient still has the same terrifying effect on me as it had the first time.

"Don't look so scared, Doc," the Captain managed to say. "This old horse isn't going to croak in your office. Just take care of me."

Of course I took care of him. And each day, in the coronary care unit, we talked. We spoke of the days at sea, of Iceland, and of Reykjavik. We reminisced about the beautiful Nordic women, so tall and striking—and who refused to have anything to do with us. And swimming in huge geyser-heated pools, constructed by the Nazis before the war.

We joked over our haphazard shipboard poker games, played on moistened tablecloths to prevent the cards from flying as the North Sea pitched our ship mercilessly. The Captain seemed to look forward to my visits as much as I did.

Despite our long talks, each day he threatened to sign himself out of the hospital, but I still had one unplayed card.

"What did you do on my ship," he kept asking me, "besides win at poker?"

"If you'll stay put, I promise to tell you. If you leave before you're well, I'll never tell you."

He survived his myocardial infarction and later underwent coronary bypass surgery. On the day he was discharged, he said, "Well, Doc, are you going to tell me now what you did on my ship?"

"Captain, I was an able seaman, and because I had finished my premedical school training, you decided to make me a pharmacist's mate."

One year later, Captain Ripchen sent me a photograph of the *Mankato Victory,* that old WWII transport ship, which now hangs over my desk as a memento of those exciting days at sea.

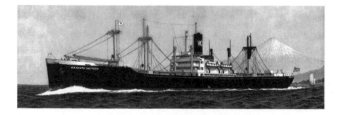

Dying to Live

Eric G. Anderson, MD

W hat's a bigamist?" Lester Teitelbaum asked me.

I grinned at him. I knew I didn't have to answer. He was going to tell me. "It's a man with one wife too many," he said. "And what's a monogamist?" he went on. I looked at his wife for inspiration. She was no help, sighing and flicking the pages of her magazine in a resigned manner.

"I don't know," I said.

"It's a man with one wife too many!" he cried, his voice cackling with amusement at his own joke.

"Lester, that's enough. Behave yourself," said Esther, his long-suffering wife, the magazine put down, a glint in her eye.

The elderly ex-accountant from Brooklyn stopped chuckling and bent over.

I pulled on a glove. I wasn't surprised to have the spouse in the room for this. Most of my geriatrics patients come two at a time like Noah's animals to the ark. Nothing I do to one seems to offend the sensitivities of the other. ECGs, pelvics, rectals—the other always stays, even occasionally takes a look. I figure they're sending me a message: if they can get through the Great Depression together, raise kids together, and still stay together, they can surely go through doctor visits together.

I bent over my patient.

"Hey, Doc, if you find a dozen roses in there, read the card for me," croaked Lester's voice from somewhere beyond my area of interest.

"Lester!" scolded his wife.

His sphincter relaxed. I checked his prostate.

I waited until he pulled on his slacks.

"There's a little area that bothers me a bit. I'd like to run a test called PSA; it stands for . . ."

". . . Pacific Southwest Airlines?"

"No, Lester. Be serious. Prostate-specific antigen. It's a fairly new marker for changes in the prostate. Both normal enlargement and tumors can raise it in the blood, but usually the test is helpful." He bounced off the table, picked up the lab test sheet, gave me a cheery wave, and took off.

His PSA result came back at about ten times normal. He saw a urologist. He had advanced cancer of the prostate.

But it was worse than that. He seemed to have lung cancer and a CNS malignancy as well. He was seen by two oncologists, then a third. It wasn't clear to any if the other two malignancies were secondary to the prostate or primary, an unusual but not impossible situation. But the questions were academic. Lester was not long for this world.

Esther went into a frenzy of activity. She wanted, of course, to understand everything. She wanted more opinions.

"This isn't a second opinion, Mrs Teitelbaum," said the last oncologist, not unkindly. "Surely it's the fourth." He then explained to both of them the futility of treatment. Mr Teitelbaum had severe diabetes mellitus and emphysema—and advanced coronary artery disease with hypertension.

She wanted referral to a major, world-famous clinic. Instead, the doctor gave the patient perhaps the best advice I've ever heard an oncologist give under the circumstances.

"Go home," he said, placing a gentle hand on Mr Teitelbaum's shoulder, "go home and spend some time with your loved ones."

It was not to be.

Lester disappeared from my care. Dropped out of sight as if he'd entered a witness-protection program. I left many messages on his answering machine.

Three weeks later he resurfaced, looking gaunt and ill. His clothes hung on him. I was astonished at how much weight he'd lost in so short a time. He tried a smile of greeting, then, with surprising difficulty, dragged a letter from the manila envelope he was carrying.

It was a summary of an extensive workup at the famous clinic. It agreed the patient was moribund but considered several heroic measures that might make a difference. I'd known my patient for years, helped him fill out his durable power of attorney for health care, and was as familiar with his choices in that matter as I was of my own. I didn't, however, want to close a door that might give him comfort. There wasn't a single suggestion in his letter that I agreed with, but I arranged for him to see our local oncologist again the next day. I felt he was entitled to that.

I was called to the hospital emergency department that night. It was Lester. I entered his cubicle as an exhausted team was trying to resuscitate him. They'd just attempted defibrillation again. "Fifth time," a nurse whispered to me. The ED doctor raised the paddles once more. "Stand back!" The patient's arms flailed up, and his head fell over towards me, pupils dilated, yet I'd swear he recognized me and gave me a smile, as if he was finally finding peace.

I stepped forward and touched the elbow of the perspiring young physician. "Stop," I murmured. "Your patient's dying. I know he wouldn't want this. He has terminal cancer. Thank you but stop. Let him be." The team drew back, relieved to have the responsibility taken from them.

"The family's here," offered the nurse. "They're in the side room. They've been in to watch."

"I'll go and see them," I said, "but fetch me out a minute later. Then I'll go back a second time with a full report. I'll use the first visit to prepare them. It's kinder that way."

I drew in a breath and went into the family room.

Inside pacing were Lester's wife, their two daughters, and a son-in-law. I nodded to the others and took the wife's hand.

With what I felt was the skill and wisdom of 30 years as a physician, I said, "You know the resuscitation team has been working on Lester. But it's not working. This illness is going to be more than he can handle. I'm going back to check him but I want you to be ready for what's probably going to be bad news . . ."

My nurse appeared in the doorway. "Doctor," she said. I turned to go. Mrs Teitelbaum grabbed my arm.

"Save him," she said, "We've canceled his living will, Lester and I. We want everything done. Keep the IVs going. Put him on a machine. I want him kept alive."

"Yes," echoed a daughter. "You must listen to our wishes. You mustn't give up."

The adversarial issues of the American legal system swam before me. I hadn't readdressed the patient's options the day before. What if the family was right? I'd stopped a code on a patient who wasn't quite dead although I felt sure rigor mortis was starting even as we spoke. Yet I'd heard of physicians who'd been sued by families for less. Lester and I had discussed his thoughts on more than one occasion—but not recently. Surely the family knew my patient's wishes better than I.

I turned to the silent daughter. "Let me check your father again. What you're telling me is critical. I can give you only a minute before I come back. When I return, you've got to clarify this. I need to know where we stand. But I've known your father's wishes for years. I know what he wanted."

I slipped away. My patient was stone dead. No respirations. No heart-beat. Pupils fixed, dilated.

I went back. If they wanted to continue resuscitation efforts, I might be in trouble. The son-in-law was speaking. "Give up, Mom," he said. "Lester told me last night—and you heard him—he didn't want to go on."

She dropped back into her seat. Her daughters sat on the arms of her chair, and all three looked up.

"He doesn't have to fight anymore, Mrs Teitelbaum," I said. "He's gone. It's over."

Esther stood up, sank her face into my chest, and wailed, "I've lost him."

"I've lost him too," I said.

She looked up with her tear-stained face and patted my cheek.

The Disability Blues

Dean Schillinger, MD

I glance at my nurse's annotation: "NEW PATIENT—H/O SUB-
STANCE ABUSE. HERE FOR DISABILITY RE-EVAL."

Mr E, a 56-year-old man, enters my examination room. To describe
him as disheveled is to oversimplify. He shuffles toward me in trash-
picked sneakers whose tongues wag for want of laces. His pants bunch at
his ankles like an accordion. Barely clinging to his hips, they drag down
his whole being. Nose to the ground, he is forced to look straight up,
past his brow and silver Afro, just to achieve eye contact. His posture
suggests a question mark. He drools, unable to counter the gravitational
pull on his lower lip. Gravity is the force that brings him to my doorstep.
He is truly down and out.

I invite him to take a seat and I wonder what will become of our interaction. Will I diagnose ankylosing spondylitis, or severe spinal degenerative joint disease? Will I obtain radiographs documenting the sorry state
of his vertebral column, and describe the resultant functional impair-
ments? Will I uncover cirrhosis or HIV infection, or find no diagnosis
other than "urban decay"—a diagnosis nobody wants to pay for? And
most of all, how will I be able to relate to this question mark of a man?

I begin our interview with the standard medical questionnaire. His
responses are marked by frequent digressions and an aggressive tone.
Our initial few minutes leave me frustrated. My frustration is obvious; he
becomes equally frustrated. Our mutual agitation crescendoes; I think I
may have to end the interview and refer him elsewhere.

Changing the tone of our conversation, I ask him what type of work
he used to do.

"Well, I played the trombone," he rasps. "Yeah . . . I played with the
greats. . . . But no more. . . . No, sir, . . . no more."

"Really?" I am stimulated, reawakened. "*I* play sax."

He responds with an edentulous, cavernous, soaring smile. "No kiddin', Doc?"

I smile a smile of polished, ivory teeth. "Well, I'm not so good, but it's still fun."

"That's cool, Doc. Real cool. Hey! I got a sax-playin' doc!"

He recounts the gigs with Bill Evans, Dizzy, Coltraine, and Miles—all those gigs, all the good times, all the girls, and he smiles and as he talks, he taps his foot to a rhythm of the past.

His smile gradually surrenders to gravity's lamenting pull downward. "But now, . . . now I got no *chops*, Doc." He tells me about the heavy drinking, the heroin, the bad times. He can't remember much after that. We talk some more—talk jazz, talk about Oakland in the '60s and '70s. He tells me about the methadone, gives me the name of his "payee" and friend at his temporary hotel.

I return to his medical history. Now he willingly shows me his laparotomy scar from "my bleedin' ulcer," and his swollen feet. He is bad with details. His short-term memory is poor. He is undoubtedly demented. I briefly examine him, order some blood work, and ask him to return in two weeks. He takes my card with the appointment time and pockets it.

As he leaves, I wonder what would have happened had we not stumbled upon this common interest. Would we have parted angrily, each cast into a stereotyped role that neither of us was comfortable fulfilling? Are racial, social, and class differences so great that only such fortuitous connections can rescue the clinical encounter? Was this good fortune, a narrow escape from the frequent failure to recognize the basic shared humanity that should sustain any therapeutic relationship?

Mr E misses his follow-up appointment. He returns four weeks later. His blood work is normal. I perform a Mini–Mental State Examination. We move at a snail's pace. He is scoring miserably. When faced with one of the final items—WRITE A SENTENCE—he takes my pen and wraps himself around the paper. I tell him to take his time, and I sit down to do my charting. A few seconds later, he reaches out and passes me the paper.

_____ Write a sentence (1 point):

I look at his face—a smile, and an unmistakable look of pride.

"What does it say?" I ask.

"Boom boom . . . diggiduh bmm-boom."

I give him a point for it.

I would like to thank Margaret Wheeler and Ariella Hyman for their editorial assistance.

Livia

Joel Lazar, MD

Grand as any goddess, three-breasted Livia, flesh tumbling forth in endless folds of inertia, you have grown into some mammoth and mythic embodiment of my fears and frustration.

I recall our first meeting: Layer upon layer of Livia piled onto a hospital stretcher, not so much gasping for air as gulping it wetly. At home you have fallen from your chair, and now the breathing pains you. Here, and here, across your broad chest, where you met the hard floor.

Years back you lost your legs to bad sugar, and no one imagined your spirit would survive that grim mutilation. But you were motion then, courage and will. You fashioned a world of idiosyncratic efficiency, leveled tables and lifted platforms to refit your home to wheelchair elevation, made possible the slow but sure transfers from bed to chair, from chair to commode, from commode to chair to bed.

But Liv, you are larger than life, and your poor arms could not carry you forever. The weight of responsibility ground your bones slowly, one into the next, and the tendons of your shoulders were torn from years of effort.

Someone gave you aspirin for those shoulders, until finally you bled so badly into your gut that only a surgeon could patch you up. Yet you would not rest your arms (how could you?), so the grinding and tearing continued. Then narcotics, which lulled your great bowels into passivity. Slower now, less sure, the transfers from bed to chair, from chair to commode, such a burden as arms were not built to bear.

And now you have fallen, for of course you must eventually fall, and a fractured rib digs into your side. You splint your breaths like some great gulping fish, and to my stethoscope there are indeed oceans inside you, rising for lack of a cough to clear them.

I lift your gown to examine, and am shocked at what is not your breast but a breast-like protrusion beneath and between the usual two:

a huge ventral hernia, your GI surgery gone bad. To my touch it has the texture of a satchel of rocks, as if months of old stool had collected there.

Painful, Ma'am? And you gulp again loudly, scowl at my prodding.

How long since your last bowel movement? But you cannot hear (this too?), not since your hearing aid dislodged and was lost forever. Swallowed up, I imagine, in rolls of impenetrable pannus. I must holler in this public place, BOWEL MOVEMENT, and you get my meaning, shake your head no.

And I apprehend, even in these first 15 minutes, the world we two shall create these next several months. Your poor life has been a series of indignities, and now you have come to share them with me, so that we may suffer indignity together.

Mornings and mornings and mornings, until something like ritual evolves from the daily litany of our failures. I must write you brief messages on a pad at your bedside. PAIN? Here and there, when I breathe. HEARING AID? Still waiting for a new one. BOWEL MOVEMENTS? Nothing, Doctor, nothing at all.

Undeterred, I Narc you and Scan you and Fleet you. Medicine is an art of linguistic transformation, simple nouns forged into phrases of action. But Livia, you are the antithesis of verb.

There is no more strength in these arms that were your legs, and your wet gulping lungs cannot support whatever Rehab those arms may require, and your mythic third breast grows full with stool when I soften with morphine the pain that stabs your wet lungs, and you cannot even hear what pity I offer you, and because you cannot hear it I begin to withhold it.

MOVING THE ARMS? Just dragging them, can't you see. AND BREATHING ANY BETTER? You cannot imagine the pain. AND ANY SUCCESS WITH THE ENEMAS? Nothing, Doctor, nothing at all.

Every organ takes its cue from the others, falls inward into your collective deceleration. Every pore of you, Livia, every cell, grinds toward a halt. Motion itself becomes mass, and I believe you are growing, if only to contain my own hyperbolic projection of defeat.

Senior physicians keep their distance. Better trained than I, they can sense failure from afar. There is wet music in your lungs that no one shall hear except me, and clay in your pendulous third breast that no one else shall feel.

Why do you leave here so quickly each morning? I STAY, LIV, AS LONG AS I CAN. When am I going home? NOT HOME, BUT ELSEWHERE.

HOW CAN YOU FEND FOR YOURSELF? I come to you sick, and you send me away sicker. THEN TELL ME . . . What? TELL ME ABOUT YOUR BOWEL MOVEMENTS.

Nothing, Doctor. Nothing at all.

Here is my life, poor old Livia, bound up in your bowels. None of us moving, neither you nor they nor I. This is why I try to pry them open. Because I am stuck inside you as well.

So much flesh, so much body, you must surely be the embodiment of something. Three-breasted Livia, perched in your bed like some ancient totem, you are goddess of failed effort, queen of stagnation.

WE HAVE FOUND YOU A NURSING HOME. I don't want to go. BUT YOU MUST. In three months this is all you have done for me? BUT LIV . . . What have you done for me Doctor: nothing.

Nothing at all.

And you fail to appreciate the great power of your cruel words, as I fail to recognize the flailing desperation in your cruelty.

The wheels of Nursing Home Placement complete their slow turn, and I do not raise a hand to stop them. My very actions, burdened by our mutual frustration, seem like a failure to act. As you cannot budge for me, Liv, neither can I budge for you. Not even when we say good-bye:

Doctor, I come to you sick . . . I KNOW YOU WILL DO WELL. You send me away . . . LIVIA . . .

. . . sicker.

Joshua Knew

Liana Roxanne Clark, MD

Joshua knew before I did that it was time. I went to see him just as I had done numerous mornings before. He lay on his bed, still, except for the slow rise and fall of his chest. His sallow skin was lined with fine blue veins. I drew closer, avoiding the tangle of tubing and wires that sprouted from him like roots from a plant. His small hands rested delicately on his distended belly. He was a small boy, appearing much younger than his 5 years. He slept peacefully, his sandy-blond, sleep-tousled hair decorating his pillow. His round cheeks were spattered with brown freckles. A clear oxygen mask covered an upturned nose and slightly agape mouth.

I nodded to his mother, who sat ever present at his bedside. As I leaned over to listen to his chest with my stethoscope, Joshua awakened. His teal blue eyes fixed on my face.

"I don't need this anymore," he said, and pulled off the oxygen mask. "I'm ready to die now."

I looked at his mother, trying to hide my shock. For three weeks I had struggled to make this child well enough to go home for what would inevitably be his last Christmas. Now, on December 17, Joshua was telling me that the fight was over. His mother reached to take his hand and I backed away from the bed. Joshua had drifted back into unconsciousness. I felt a lump forming in my throat, and I knew that tears would soon follow.

As I left the room, I struggled to regain control of my emotions. I had felt so helpless, standing by, watching Joshua die, bit by bit, unable to heal him. Looking through his hospital room window, I saw his mother speaking to him, pausing to kiss him softly on the forehead. She seemed so strong, while I felt as if I were being torn apart.

As I turned away, I saw Joshua's father walking toward the room. I leaned back heavily against the wall, as if seeking strength from the building itself. Covered with the faces of gaily colored smiling clowns, the wall was a stark contrast to my solemn expression. He approached me, searching my face for some sign of hope. Slowly, I managed to form the words, to tell him that Joshua was ready to die. He set his jaw grimly and went inside. I followed reluctantly.

Both parents now stood next to him. They murmured softly, telling him how much they loved him. I stood at a short distance, willing myself not to cry. I turned to watch the monitor, focusing intently on the tiny tracings. Gradually as I watched, the heartbeat became slower and slower, until it stopped. His parents held Joshua as they cried in their grief. Mechanically I moved forward, put the stethoscope in my ears, placed the diaphragm on Joshua's chest, and listened to the silence. He was gone.

I mumbled condolences to the parents and hurried from the room. Walking rapidly down the hall, looking neither right nor left, finally I reached the stairwell. After closing the door behind me, I sat heavily on the concrete steps. A soft wail emanated from some place deep within me. Warm tears began to flow down my cheeks as I wept quietly for Joshua. Soon, however, angry sobs racked my body as all the frustration and impotence overwhelmed me. After a while, I could cry no longer. So I sat, tracing patterns on the dusty stair, asking myself the unanswerable questions.

Why couldn't I have saved my little Joshua?

Why does AIDS have to win every time?

Thank God I Have Cancer

David M. Mumford, MD

As physicians, we eventually attain an age of reflection and solitary games. Among these mind machinations is "Memory as Lottery," an ongoing game of chance. Some thoughtful questions also arise at this stage of life: Does suffering serve any purpose? What truths have I retained in my aging residue? Now that I look back, I find my few shining grains of wisdom frequently came from patient encounters. One unassuming patient and his spouse were unknowingly indelible mentors to me. The process of dying is surely the greatest lesson plan we all must confront. To mutate a thought of Tolstoy, every death is the same, yet each is an individual human drama in which patient and caregivers play teaching roles. Sometimes the physician benefits most from these important interchanges.

In the late 1960s and early 1970s, cancer immunology was blossoming. Novel ideas were erupting; exciting new approaches were fashioned; and promised "breakthroughs" regularly floated. As part of my research, I worked in the hospital's cancer pavilion, toting a bag of immunotherapy hopes. My immune nostrums were applied randomly and included immune adjuvants, altered antigens, and rarely "hyperimmune" serum. However, tumor vaccines made from self, foreign, or cultured tissue were always a component. One winter evening I entered the fluorescently lit hospital room of an out-of-state patient admitted that morning. As I introduced myself, he was sitting stoically on the bed. His expression revealed the fatigued lines of a hesitant, but experienced, veteran of waiting. Rather slight of build and middle-aged, he was still dressed in street clothes worn for a last-minute, perhaps precautionary, stop at a nearby church. His referral letter described the failed surgery/chemotherapy treatment given for stage IV melanoma. Our medical strategy was early immunotherapy after hyperthermic perfusion of his cancer-riddled leg.

We began to talk and his passive demeanor slowly evaporated. I soon learned he was no pussy cat. A calm-appearing man, he had come to fight cancer. No offered regimen, regardless of pain or difficulty, dampened his fortitude. Indeed, some of the immune insults he endured would have elicited spontaneous applause from the Marquis de Sade. Because his skin was very fair, thin, and unusually fragile, constantly removing small tumor masses (for tumor vaccine preparations) was a repeated travail. He particularly hated the gigantic (up to one third of his back) cross-hatched BCG scarifications frequently administered. Thus, most of his days and many nights were filled with multiple injections, IVs, incisions, biopsies, and deliberate abrasions.

We soon discovered these procedures were inflicted on a man whose previous nickname, "The Swooner," was well deserved and accepted by him. "There are sensitive nervous systems, supersensitive nervous systems, and then mine," he declared. "I have developed syncope into an art form not seen since the late 19th century. I probably shouldn't tell you this, but I even fainted during my inaugural speech at my present job." Needless to say, we modified many procedures so that they could be given while he was prone! Otherwise, his self-control was exemplary. On rare occasions expletives came forth, but these were always self-directed, as if to combat a personal weakness. I knew he was glad to see me leave on "therapy" days, but we both looked forward to conversational evenings discussing life, religion, science, the healing power of humor combined with country music, and his erroneous judgment about the inferiority of Texas fishing.

Despite a flood of friends, his quiet and centered wife was the premier nurturer and gyroscope. She was always in his room, and staff called her his "care angel." One day as I entered, the room was unusually dark. She was not at the bedside and I searched the gloom until I recognized the figure on a stool in a far corner, facing the wall. Her husband was sleeping fitfully. Without turning she said, "He should be waking soon. If you are wondering why I'm sitting here, it is to give him pleasure. He says that he has lost control over everything in his life."

Then she added, "When we disagree, and we sometimes still argue, he may order me to the corner. We both know it's a macabre charade, but I go there happily and so restore a smidgen of his lost power.

"After all, it's the least I can do."

Some two months later, it was obvious his was not to be a gentle closing. Life's clock was now counting in days, and his misery intensified. I often wondered whether the additional pain and distress of immunotherapy was worth his suffering. He did live three standard deviations beyond our estimate, which encouraged the doctors. Although quality-of-life advocates might question the experimental regimen, ultimately he answered my concerns.

One afternoon I happened to visit while his wife was on an important search—an M&Ms' errand of chocolate mercy. I settled into the chair next to his bed as he turned toward me.

"David," he began, "let me tell you something. I've been imagining how it would be if my coming death were caused by a stroke, heart attack, or some other abrupt ending. When I do, I thank God I have cancer."

He paused a moment and explained. "Without this extra time, I never would have known what love and tenderness are possible between people on this earth."

I knew a profound new question challenged me: Is love the essential marrow of our humanness? I also realized an unknown door in the human spirit—one I could never glimpse through scientific reasoning—had opened to me. Suffering, however difficult, can be a wise parent to personal meaning. One person's verities may unexpectedly differ from another's. And, more enduringly, demonstrations of wisdom and grace by patients can reverberate endlessly in caregivers.

Certainly that happened to me.

The Delivery

L. Stewart Massad, MD

In the jeweled morning light of the solarium, she sat alone, combing out her thick black hair. I had not seen her before with her hair loose, such beauty and vitality spilling down her shoulders and I, with the smell of formalin still about me, was suddenly speechless with the horror of what I had come to say.

She did not seem to suspect why I had come, though we had been waiting two days for the verdict the pathologist had just given me. As her oncologist, I came to talk of cancer, yet she smiled and said hello as calmly as if we were only old acquaintances meeting again across a cafe table. I sat on the arm of a recliner, my hands in my lap. She had been looking out at the springtime, at the men and women coatless on the sidewalks, at the wind ruffling the new grass. I stared at dust motes suspended in great blocks of sunshine that struck through the wavy glass of the tall windows. Now she gazed at me, bemused by my confusion, and waited for what I had to say.

Of course, I had known the biopsy result all along. Perhaps some of her symptoms might have been written off as complications of the radiation she'd received, and that possibility was what I'd focused on, to keep hope alive. But when she'd first walked into my examining room, I had read her diagnosis in her stoop, for she carried the tumor growing inside her like a child, her hands on her belly, protective of her pain. Her bleeding, the reek of her fistula, the gritty texture of the ulcer that had been the roof of her vagina wall were typical. Viewing her radiograph, seeing the nodules that speckled her lungs, I'd felt such a catch in my own chest. Still, it is one thing to know, another to prove, and I had waited until I had seen for myself the blithe malignancy of her cancer magnified under glass before telling her.

It is the physician's job to be death's herald. Some do it badly, others less so; none do it well. There are many styles of delivering bad news.

One is the bluff pronouncement before the back turns, as if the patient bore responsibility for failure the physician cannot face. Another's the evasive approach, the doctor dancing with euphemisms until the patient catches on, insight and despair illuminate the face, and the two move on to discuss palliation, the ultimate prognosis unspoken but understood. Some try the chummy routine, death and the patient's terror belittled as only bumps along a road, to be ridden over and passed by. Sympathy can soften the jolt of knowing, but dying is a journey one travels alone; therapeutic touch and a gentle voice go only so far. Then there is the heroic exposition, death yet another challenge for physicians and patients to conquer together. Finally, the offhand mention in the office: an intimation of death left in the patient's heart like an assassin's knife.

Delivering a prognosis of mortality is no less a skill than delivering a child. It is a painful skill, one some never learn, never try to acquire, leaving their patients to discover death alone. I have never mastered it. I suspect I never will, any more than I will master death itself. Still, I try, because the door I close on hope opens to grief, accommodation, acceptance, and reconciliation.

When I could not face this woman any longer, I looked away and said, "The biopsy's back."

"Ah," she replied. "I wondered why you'd come, and with that look. And the result?"

I forced myself to look into her face. I saw trust and, perhaps, foreknowledge, since I had told her before that recurrence would be incurable, and she understood that what made her feel so bad could not be good.

"The biopsy," I told her, "is positive."

"Positive," she echoed. Her forehead furrowed. "But tell me: how can a result be positive when it means I'm going to die?"

I was ready for tears. I knew how to cope with anger, silence, denial, remonstrance, repudiation. I had faced all of those reactions before, devised and applied therapeutic solutions. But I was unprepared for dignity. Her face softened as she saw my distress, and her returning smile cut me like a turned scalpel. Her apparent acceptance accentuated my sense of helplessness; her calm deepened my despair. I couldn't answer.

It was she who roused me, asking that we move on to the distraction of action: "What now?"

I reviewed the choices: chemotherapy or observation, additional radiation to arrest the bleeding, surgery to palliate the fistula. I spoke of the efficacy of narcotics in relieving pain, the variety of the pharmacopoeia that can deny cancer some of its terror. Relieved to speak of concrete things and so evade thoughts of their ultimate futility, I went on and on, not noticing at first that her smile was gone and her eyes were no longer on me. Instead, she watched the little figures four stories down cross the green lawn between the nursing school and the park. When she did not reply to my enthusiasm, I pointed out that she had many choices to make, but none that needed to be made that day.

Without turning back, she reached for my fingers, her touch as delicate as the spring outside. "Yes," she said. "Thank you."

Her handclasp was my dismissal, but I did not go. Something still seemed unsaid. "If there's anything I can do . . ." I offered, but that wasn't it.

"I appreciate all you've done," she said, and I realized that for her what I'd done seemed at that moment no more positive than the biopsy. "But if you don't mind, I'd like to cry alone."

I realized what a fool I'd been. I had hurt her, and in my own pain I had not seen how much. "I'm sorry," I said: the words I had forgotten. She nodded, forgiving. A smile crossed her face, as subtle and as fleeting as cloud shadows on the campus below.

I thought to stay and grieve with her. But there would be time for that, and staying to watch her weep would have stripped her of the only thing cancer had not taken: her pride. I hastened away before the first tears could leak through the walls of her courage.

The Bard in His Outcast State

Steve Schlozman, MD

When Raymond first arrived at the mental health center, he looked a little like Charles Manson. He stared at me with wild, unblinking blue eyes, his hair well beyond his shoulders, his beard expanding exponentially as it made its way from his boyish face. I had heard that he was from the West, and judging from the wrinkles and sunburn that painted his face, I could easily imagine him wandering small, sleepy, dusty towns, stopping occasionally for bad coffee in tired truck stops, sometimes giggling, usually left to himself. He had spent already a good month at the state hospital, having been committed there after an arrest in one of Boston's most fashionable neighborhoods. According to his records, he had been resting on the doorstep of an expensive apartment building eating a bagel when one of the apartment's residents asked him to leave. He became violent and incoherent, yelling something about angels and how cruel they could be, and when the police arrived, in the midst of his assault on one of the police officers, he pleaded with them to see that he needed hospitalization. A familiar request from Raymond, his wish was granted, and he found himself at the state hospital receiving medications for his latest manic episode. After his spending a month there, the courts felt he no longer required the restrictions of a hospital under Department of Corrections jurisdiction, and he was subsequently transferred to a Department of Mental Health facility for further treatment. These were the events that conspired to allow Raymond and the mental health center to make an acquaintance.

His medical record was remarkable. He had a greater than 30-year history of very bad bipolar disorder, and he had been hospitalized more than 25 times. He told me with a smile, in his slightly Western accent, that he had seen and had been treated in almost every state in "our great country." Sure enough, I had received copies of his discharge summaries from seven states throughout the nation. When I noted from the chronology of his records that he had only recently wandered East, he smiled and seemed altogether honest for the first time. "That rocky, foggy coast," he said, almost dreaming. "I sure do love it in the summer. Not sure I've seen anything more beautiful, to tell you the truth." For a moment I was lost myself, remembering my own times in the North Woods.

Raymond was born in the rural part of his Western state, one of several children to whom he described as "a cruel but loving father and a timid mother." At the age of 3 he discovered a penchant for classical music, and by age 6 he was something of a prodigy, performing piano concertos throughout small towns that his father wandered with his family. Raymond lowered his voice when his father was mentioned, as if talking normally might continue to incur the wrath he grew up fearing. He told me with an uncharacteristic lack of emotion that he had been homeless for 25 years, and he brightened considerably as he began to praise the virtues of living without roots. He described for me the red rock canyons in Utah and the crashing waves of the Pacific. Though I had been to most of the places he mentioned, sitting there in the dreary confines of the mental health center, the cloudy northeastern sky providing little warmth or comfort on that late November day, I found myself gently appreciating a red-golden sunset over sparkling waters, thankful for that brief moment of freedom from my well-bounded life.

I liked Raymond and looked forward to morning rounds and to the times he and I spent talking alone. He wore flannel shirts and torn blue jeans, and when he had collected enough money from his Social Security checks, he purchased a $100 pair of walking shoes. "Gonna be discharged soon," he said, smiling. "Gotta be ready to hit the streets." He seemed torn between the comforts of a warm bed and his genuine need to keep moving. Often when we talked, he would rock in his chair or cross his legs, incessantly shaking his right foot. When I commented that his near-constant motion might suggest an adverse effect of his medications, he looked angry but sounded hurt. "This shaking," he said, "this shaking is part of me. It's who I am. When are you people gonna realize that?" Perhaps his most characteristic gesture was the furious way he would tilt his head and scratch his greasy hair with his right forefinger. This action usually heralded one of his many declarations of indisputable truths. Once, for example, upon hearing another patient's request for increased privileges denied, he looked thoughtful for a moment and then asked me whether I had heard of Nietzsche. "A smart, smart man," he said knowingly, "but he didn't believe in angels."

As Raymond's discharge date loomed nearer, he became less playful and more melancholy. The times that he and I met alone also became more volatile, with Raymond often raising his voice at the notion of his need for medications or for a financial payee. Once he and I spent an entire hour discussing the recent assassination of Yitzhak Rabin. He was obsessed with the fact that "Rabin's own people" had committed the murder. Raymond scratched his head furiously and scowled, "They act like they care, but they don't." We sat quietly for a moment, and then I asked him whether he felt that we were forcing him out of the hospital. He got up and left the room without a word.

The plan for Raymond gradually took shape, and we informed him of our intent to fly him to Tucson. He had asked earlier whether this might be possible, and he referred us to a bank account there where he thought he might have enough money for the flight. His lability continued, but he gradually began to express an almost boyish excitement at his imminent ride on an airplane. He told me of his intent to "resume the study of angels," and one morning he approached the treatment team with a request for money to buy books. "What books?" I asked, and he replied mischievously, "Oh, you know, the usual. Chaucer, Blake, Shakespeare." He mentioned that he already had the complete works of Shakespeare, and later I asked him whether he had a favorite play. "You know, I've always liked *Hamlet*," he said. "There's that whole oedipal thing, and I think Hamlet was a little manic." His hand was busily scratching his head, and he moved his right foot so fast I felt my own feet getting tired. "What about the sonnets?" I asked. "Do you have a favorite sonnet as well?" He mumbled that he knew a few of them, and I worried that my curiosity might be ill-placed. Still, when he fell silent, I decided to tell him that I had a favorite, and I recited the opening line.

"When, in disgrace with fortune and men's eyes," I began.

His hand dropped from his head. He stopped moving his foot, and looking at my feet he almost whispered, "I all alone beweep my outcast state."

"And trouble deaf heaven with my bootless cries," I continued.

"And look upon myself, and curse my fate," he said more forcefully.

And so we continued, alternating lines, growing more rhythmic in our recital, both of us sensing the other's reluctance to reach the 14th and final line. When we did finish, he smiled at me and admitted, "Yeah, I like that one too, Doc. Are we done now?" And he got up from his chair and walked slowly out of the interview room.

29

When, in disgrace with fortune and men's eyes,
I all alone beweep my outcast state,
And trouble deaf heaven with my bootless cries,
And look upon myself, and curse my fate,
Wishing me like to one more rich in hope,
Featured like him, like him with friends possessed,
Desiring this man's art and that man's scope,
With what I most enjoy contented least;
Yet in these thoughts myself almost despising,
Haply I think on thee—and then my state,
Like to the lark at break of day arising
From sullen earth, sings hymns at heaven's gate;
   For thy sweet love remembered such wealth brings
   That then I scorn to change my state with kings.

Colors

Fred Leonard, MD

More than the chill in the air, more than the shortening days, more than the echoing calls of migrating geese, there was one sure sign that winter was imminent—ski racks. Well before the first snows ever touched the Rocky Mountains, some primal force compelled the residents of Denver, Colorado, to mount ski racks on their cars, just as it compelled the Canada geese to fly south.

But there was no ski rack on my car. I was beyond noticing the changes around or in me. Besides, I just didn't have time. I had become preoccupied and absorbed by the demands of a rotating internship. Chronically sleep deprived, perennially behind, and feeling more than a little overworked, neither I nor my circadian rhythms seemed to be able to adjust to the unremitting routine of every second and every third night call. Now, five months into this 12-month ordeal, I had completed my obstetric and surgical rotations and had started ward medicine—a tedious and joyless service that was viewed by all but the most zealous among us as penance for any stimulation or fulfillment that we might otherwise salvage from the rest of the internship year.

Outside the medicine wards, the November days had continued to shorten. As daylight became little more than a dim memory, I found myself living in a colorless rod-vision-gray world, illuminated only by the stark fluorescent fixtures of the hospital and the cold mercury-vapor street lamps that cut through the darkness of my morning and evening commutes. I no longer even saw the sun rise or set. But, as a fellow intern pointed out, it hardly mattered. After all, there was nothing beautiful about a sunrise if you were too bleary-eyed to focus on it.

Populating my colorless, gray world were the gray-haired ward medicine patients. We interns all knew that somewhere outside the confines of the hospital lurked the Supreme Nursing Home Triage Officer. It was his duty to ensure that every night on call we each received at least one demented, aphasic patient with a chief complaint of "won't eat," "less responsive," or "no bowel movement for two weeks." Then for the ensuing days, weeks, and months of our ward medicine rotations (and we feared it could become years), we visited these poor souls twice daily on ward rounds—a monotonous ritual that seemed to reflect the dearth of vitality and spontaneity that so characterized us, our mentors, and our surroundings.

So it was with no sense of joy or adventure that particular night on call that I trudged toward the emergency department for my third admission of the evening. As I wandered down the fluorescent-lit corridors, I tried to calculate how many hours of sleep debt I had accrued to that point in my internship. My calculations were still incomplete when the ED nurse pointed me toward the curtained cubicle containing my new patient. There, with an IV in her left arm and leaning over a stainless steel emesis basin, was Carol. She appeared pale, fatigued, and acutely ill, but in-between her retching and rapid respirations she managed to acknowledge my presence with a weak smile. Carol was being admitted with a diagnosis of diabetic ketoacidosis.

Having learned at least something from five months as an intern, I rapidly assessed the situation. Here was a patient who was about my age, could talk, had an acute clinical problem, and had not come from a nursing home. Maybe there had been a mistake. Maybe I had gone into the wrong cubicle. Maybe the Supreme Nursing Home Triage Officer was temporarily indisposed. It didn't matter. She was my patient now. Before anyone could correct the obvious error, I pushed gurney, IV, emesis basin, and Carol out of the ED and up to the wards.

By morning, both Carol and I were still tired but feeling better—she because her metabolic derangements were coming under control, and I because I now had a patient whom I looked forward to seeing on rounds. Not only was she my first patient with diabetic ketoacidosis, she was my first ward medicine patient with whom I could carry on a "normal" conversation.

Over the next few days, I spent as much time as I could talking with Carol. She had what we then called juvenile-onset diabetes. The term fit well, for diabetes had taken control of her life when she was just 12 years old. Now, 19 years later, it had also taken her eyesight, robbed her of sensation in her feet, and was well on its way to claiming her kidneys. Yet she was cheerful, upbeat, and thankful for what she had been allowed to do in her life. When she began to lose her vision two years before, she had learned to read Braille, and she planned to help others do the same. She knew she would soon be on dialysis, yet she accepted its inevitability and was hopeful that she would be a candidate for a kidney transplant. She had only one small regret. That fall she had been in the Rockies, and though she could feel their grandeur and beauty, she could no longer see their striking yellow aspens or rugged green landscape and azure sky. She truly longed to see the colors of a Rocky Mountain fall just one more time.

I did not tell Carol I had missed the aspens that fall. Being too busy, too immersed, too overwhelmed hardly seemed an adequate excuse. How could I tell her I had not seen those brilliant fall colors simply because I had not made an effort to open my eyes? After a mere five months of internship, I had become jaded and unseeing, with neither the time nor the inclination to experience the overwhelming beauty of life. Diabetes had taken Carol's eyesight. Internship had apparently taken mine.

Carol went home after four days in the hospital, and she was not re-admitted during my internship year. As with most of my patients from that year, I never saw her again. Yet her effect on me and my internship did not end with her discharge. Though the call schedules, the demands, and the dehumanizing routines did not change, my perspectives slowly did. Both inside and outside the hospital, I began to notice the ever-present life, light, and colors. I even found that I could talk with my gray-haired patients, and they had much to teach me if I just made the effort to listen. And I have never since missed seeing the colors of fall. Nor has a fall passed that I have not thought of Carol, the person who helped me see them.

Cristina

Peggy Hansen, MD

The flesh has melted from her, mere wax beneath the flame of the rapacious tumor living in her pelvis. She's a frequent flyer, one of those patients who returns for many visits, and we know her well. They come back to have tubes checked or changed, to have more tubes inserted, or to have a tube removed, and with each visit they are somehow changed. For most, it is a subtle thing, perhaps a little weight loss or a faint new line across a weathered forehead. For Cristina, though, there is no missing it: she has become, in the span of one short month, a listless vestige of the woman we last saw.

She has cervical cancer, and she is here with us because the mass has risen like a greedy neighbor and laid claim to territory not its own. It has shut down her kidneys with an unmoving roadblock, and we have put tubes in through her back to carry out the urine and restore their function. They are her lifeline now, these slender tubes, and her husband cares for them with due respect, calling us with questions or progress reports. He is diligent and careful, qualities too scarce in this embattled world, and he loves her in a fierce and tender way. His expression, the set of his jaw, tell me he would gladly call out death and challenge it, if only death would answer him.

Because I am an interventional radiologist, my desire and my training are to intervene, to do things that will fix a problem. In this regard my practice is like surgery, although it is done without the use of large incisions or bulky metal tools. Some days I am like a happy plumber, delving into blockages and coming up with bits of stone pulled from the depths to show the grateful patient. Other days I am less sanguine, knowing there is little I can do to help the person lying on my table: no mere plumbing problem, this, but a cracked foundation well beyond my powers.

There is no intervening left for Cristina, none that will do her any good, at least. She is "maxed out" on treatment: she has had it all, none of it effective, and she can get no more. Neither chemotherapy nor radiation has assuaged the beast, and so we wait for it to finish her. It is not easy, this waiting, for her or for us. No matter how many times it is repeated, this is a heartless lesson, and one that all of us in medicine find difficult to handle. Many deal with it by outright denial, a stubborn refusal to believe we could ever be so powerless. Others are more realistic, but no less impassioned. We see the same resistance in our patients, and in their families too, urging us to "just try *something.*" Together we grasp at the thinnest straws on which a life might hang, hoping *this* case will somehow be the one to break free of past histories and failures.

This desperation is a fairly recent thing, a product of advances in technology and science that allowed us to expect more from our medicine. No one wants to hear, these days, that death is part of life, that it comes indeed for all of us at one time or another. And no one wants to hear that doing nothing may at times be kinder than doing something, kinder than any gift of false hope and cruel expectation. So we go on, offering more chemotherapy or radiation, more surgeries or other interventions, and sometimes I wonder who it is that we are treating so heroically. We fight even more persistently when the patient is young and the disease is harsh, when the patient is someone like Cristina.

Having known Cristina makes me want to run out in the street and grab the arms of women passing by: I want to yell at them to get their Pap smears, to go see their doctors, or go to the clinic and get it done, just get it done, for pity's sake! Or, sometimes, I want to shake their husbands or their boyfriends, tell them if you love these women then you make them get it done. But of course I never do. Such passion scares us: there is something frightening about zealotry, even when we are in complete agreement, something that is unattractive and disturbing. Faced with such intemperance, we recoil, shake our heads reprovingly, and walk away as quickly as seems decent, hoping that we have remained untainted. So I keep them to myself, these fantasy crusades along the streets of Dallas, and try not to think of Cristina too often. She was only 40.

The Little Picture

Barry Gelman, MD

By now, she had earned the label "miracle child."

One of our oldest survivors with congenital HIV infection, this 7-year-old's medical history was almost legendary. Even the greenest of interns knew of Kyneisha, the little AIDS girl with more lives than the luckiest cat. She had survived numerous bouts of pneumonia, three episodes of severe respiratory failure, recurrent bacterial tracheitis, and months of hospitalization. She underwent tracheostomy. She suffered pneumothoraces. She experienced withdrawal and prolonged weakness after lengthy courses of narcotics and muscle relaxants. High PEEP meant nothing to her. Shock was just slightly bothersome. Malnutrition was a way of life. More than once, the PICU staff had told her mother that death was imminent. That treatment was approaching futility. That she should consider withdrawal of care. That we wanted to quit.

And then, she would get better. Without providing any clear understanding of how or why, she would recover. And not just a little. No matter how sick she was, each time she would eventually recover to baseline and be discharged. Home. Back to school. Back to her family and friends. Back to her idea of a regular life.

These were my thoughts as I made my way to the emergency department to see her. Maybe this would be a false alarm. She was supposedly doing so well. Maybe the ED resident was panicking over nothing.

One glance at Kyneisha was all I needed. Tachypnea. Air hunger. Cyanosis. The look of apprehension on her face. As I held her hand and tried to console her, my mind was rapidly predicting the future. Dense bilateral infiltrates. Hypotension. Fever. The ventilator. Central lines. Pancytopenia. Days, maybe weeks in the ICU.

With all that would come the inevitable questions. "Why are you being so aggressive?" "Don't you realize she's suffering?" "What kind of life does she have?" The questions come from all directions. From residents. From nurses. From Quality Assurance. From ethics rounds. From visiting professors. From colleagues. And from me. I could hear my own mind shouting at me: "Is this cost-effective?" "Who's paying for it?" "What about the waste of limited resources?" "Don't you know she's going to die, regardless?" "Think of the big picture!" "Don't you know the big picture?"

Days later, I find myself at Kyneisha's bedside. She is stable now. She is motionless, except for the rhythmic rise and fall of her chest. Her pharmacologic coma prevents her from speaking, but words are unnecessary. The soft hum of the ventilator, the blinking lights of the monitor, the slow drip of formula through her nasogastric tube, the warmth of her skin—they all remind us that she is still here, struggling, fighting to keep going. Occasionally, a solitary tear emerges from her eye and falls gently to her pillow.

There have been many tears. Too many for one so young, some would say. But there have also been the smiles. Smiles. Laughter. Moments of discovery. The joy she brings to those around her. Brief glimpses of a real childhood. Perhaps these should be the true measure of her quality of life, not the number of hospital days. Impossible amidst such a dismal existence? Not at all. Not if you know Kyneisha. Images from her past admissions fill my memory. I can remember her triumphantly clutching her teddy bear as her muscle relaxants were wearing off. I recall the delightful anticipation as she sampled her first french fry after weeks of tube feedings. I remember her flashing that shy grin while being wheeled out of the ICU to her regular room.

Those moments seem far away, now that Kyneisha is critical again. Her mother, with almost no emotion left to muster, has been through it all before. Treatises about opportunistic organisms. Daily blood cultures. Myriad ventilator adjustments. The rationale for sedation and paralysis. Painful discussions about DNR. And she keeps coming. Every day and every night. And the nurses continue caring for Kyneisha. So do the respiratory therapists and social workers and child life specialists and most everyone else. Why? Why spend so much time, energy, and money caring for a child who may die tomorrow?

Because tomorrow is hope. Because tomorrow can be filled with joy and wonder. Tomorrow can be a trip to Disney World. Or another Christmas morning. Or a birthday party. Or a few more french fries. Or a grasp of a teddy bear. Or a shy grin that brightens the entire room.

Tomorrow can be another day in a precious, little life.

How can we ascertain what that day is worth? What units should we use to quantitate what another day could mean to Kyneisha and her loved ones? Who are we to judge?

And so they continue. Mom and the nurses and the respiratory therapists and the social workers and the play therapists and the chaplains and secretaries and everyone else. None of them is ready to quit, because they know Kyneisha isn't ready to quit. Not today, anyway.

I know the big picture.

I also know Kyneisha.

I'm not ready to quit either.

Kyneisha died in hospice, the morning of July 8, 1994.—ED.

Until the Peppers

Bernadine Z. Paulshock, MD

Most people think of Delaware as an industrialized state, albeit a small one. As a matter of fact, agriculture is still Delaware's main source of revenue. And where there is agriculture, there are farmworkers, many of them seasonal or, as they are less gracefully but more descriptively called, migrants. Migrant farmworkers are now almost always residents of the United States, if not yet citizens. They are legal immigrants, perambulating farmworkers by vocation, in part because that is the only work they know and in part because it does not require a higher education or knowledge of English.

One summer some years ago, perhaps 15, my boss and my conscience coerced me into working two evenings a month at a clinic for migrant workers in southern Delaware. The building had once been a school and was now a "community center," on its way to something more lucrative, I was sure. It was drab and rundown and ill-equipped to be a medical facility. The clinic's funding paid for the rent, a few, minimal supplies, a van to pick up the workers, and some nursing and director salaries. We physicians—faculty and staff from a family practice residency in Wilmington—worked free.

Back then migrant farmworkers were often imported just for the season. Many spoke Spanish, but there were a few from French (Creole)–speaking Haiti. Most patients were young children with runny noses or abraded knees and no record of immunizations. The lollipop we gave them at the end of their visits may have been the real reason they came to the clinic, if that's what you can call a couple of little rooms in a basement. There was no sink, no examining table. Our equipment was our own sphygmomanometers, otoscopes, and stethoscopes.

The adults were mostly illiterate, even in their own languages, and most were previously uncared for. Except for the few who were truly ill, most seemed doubtful that much good would come from their seeing the doctor, especially one who could not speak their language. And they did not want to be told not to work, for if they didn't work they didn't get paid.

One August evening my patients included an old woman from Haiti. Well, she wasn't really that old since she was my age, still in her 40s. That was part of what was so shocking to me. She looked a generation older: many absent teeth, scraggly hair, torn and dingy clothes, dispirited attitude. Yet at the neck of her faded blouse was a brooch with "pearls" and brilliants, half of them missing. She did not speak English.

At least I could practice a few words of French, I thought. But I found my easiest phrases were more adapted to things like "Encore un plus du vin, s'il vous plaît" or "Je me préfère mon homard avec beurre noire au lieu de mayonnaise" than to the interchanges of a patient encounter. Still, I examined her carefully and tried to take a decent history. Her complaint was "douleur à l'arriéré de ma tête" ("pain in the back of my head"), which made sense to me inasmuch as her blood pressure was about 280/150. She was able to communicate that she had been told before her blood pressure was high but that now she had "ne pas des pilules" ("no pills"). Some years ago she had a supply for a few days, perhaps it was two summers ago. The pills had been prescribed in some other migrant worker clinic, I bet myself, and I sat back to think what to do about her.

Our clinic had a minipharmacy of a few pharmaceutical staples. For hypertension we had some hydrochlorothiazide tablets. In my own practice, a new patient with blood pressure as high as hers and with symptoms might have been hospitalized, and certainly would have been subjected to a battery of tests before or concomitant with prescribing.

But how could I perform those tests here? I decided I would have to prescribe without benefit of studies of any sort and then follow-up with several more visits to see if my therapy worked, or plan something else if it did not. Were there laboratory tests available? A BUN or creatinine? A blood glucose? Perhaps a few basics, such as an ECG?

The clinic director seemed unhappy at my request. There might be a way to do some tests if they were absolutely necessary, but they would have to be paid for out of the director's meager funds, she said. Her concern was evident and well founded: At the very least the patient would be pulled from the fields for the tests; the field boss might become angry or refuse to cooperate. The director hoped I wouldn't go overboard.

All this only strengthened my conviction that all I could do was treat my patient empirically with hydrochlorothiazide and see how she responded. How much time did I have? I wondered. I hoped to have her blood pressure under control before she returned to Haiti.

"How long will you be here?" I asked her, my pocket calendar in hand.

"Jusqu'à les poivrons," she replied. Until the peppers.

Her three words in French shocked me at the same time they made me sad and angry. For me, they were the stuff of which campaigners for better health care are made. Her answer changed me, made me uncomfortable about our "clinic." Was it in fact a charade and not worth our time? Adequate care requires continuity of facility if not of therapist. Such a frequent problem as hypertension cannot be evaluated and treated in one visit, or without tests, or without medicines. Washing a child's abraded knee does not absolve a health team from the responsibility of knowing that immunizations are up-to-date, or have been given at all.

I wondered when the peppers would be harvested, then realized they are warm-weather vegetables and knew my patient would not be returning to the clinic for very many more visits, if at all. In that moment my patient taught me that a few summer evenings in a makeshift clinic with volunteer physicians and no other resources would never satisfy the unmet needs of the truly poor, be they migrants or permanent residents. Something more was needed.

Then as now, the debate about whether health care was a right or a privilege was being vigorously argued. But that evening I understood that the "pepper lady"—with her family harvesting the melons and tomatoes and other vegetables for my table—was entitled to access to adequate health care while she was here, and at her next location and the next.

Now, 15 years later, there is still a clinic for farm workers in southern Delaware, but it is in a better building and the examination rooms are greatly improved. Still operating under the aegis of the Delmarva Rural Ministries, it receives US Public Health Service migrant health center dollars; its funding has not been increased in four years. The clinic now participates in a national computerized system that keeps track of, at least in theory, the immunizations migrant children receive. In fact, the Delaware clinic is now developing its own immunization tracking system. The physician staff is still made up of volunteers from the community.

From time to time, I wonder if adequate access will ever become a reality for all. And, after all these years, but especially during the season when

Delaware crops are in the farmers' markets, I wonder what happened to the "pepper lady" and if she ever got treatment for her hypertension before it killed her.

Heartpains

Joseph K. Izes, MD

I was slowly developing a distaste for Wednesday PGY-1 medical clinic. Every week I was stumped as I searched for medical interventions that would work in the face of insurmountable social problems. A 400-pound housekeeper was upset that anti-inflammatory drugs were not helping her low back pain. An entire family of Cambodian refugees, unable to communicate in English or any mutually understandable gestures, still mystified me. I could feel my carefully groomed synaptic pathways, my algorithms of differential diagnosis and therapeutics, beginning to decay. Each Wednesday evening, my thoughts were as tangled as my thinning hair, occasionally pulled out at the roots by my tugging.

Even more disturbing was the talent I was developing in quickly satisfying the concerns of these patients. Only rarely was I able to make a precise diagnosis and recommend a reliable remedy. Yet somehow they left the office renewed, hopefully clutching their prescriptions and dutifully making their follow-up appointments. It bothered me to be so over-appreciated when, by my own standards, I accomplished so little. There was no science here.

My last new patient of the day was waiting. Her record was thick and overflowed its flimsy cardboard binder. Scanning the illegible scrawl of ten years of interns, who apparently felt the same way I did about the medical clinic, was unenlightening. She had been treated for high blood pressure in the past. A brief salvo of unusual chest pains started the usual medical investigations, and a mild antianginal agent had been prescribed. There were many visits for no discernible reason. While vital signs were documented, no clear complaint, symptoms, or physical findings were recorded. These seemed to be almost social visits with no specific diagnosis or treatment noted in the chart.

She had not been to the clinic for two years. Apparently a zealous intern had elicited the fact that she constantly heard music. She was surprised that the doctor did not. The music was beautiful and did not frighten her. The last entry in the chart was a request for a psychiatric consultation. That appointment had never been kept.

I entered the examination room and had to look around to find the small, elderly woman sitting on my low rolling stool in the far corner. She did not acknowledge my presence.

I glanced at the chart again—she was 82 years old and lived alone in one of the seedier parts of town. She wore a faded print housedress, an overcoat, galoshes, and a brightly patterned kerchief on her head. Her face was wrinkled, her eyes were bright blue and very watery. She seemed upset.

I introduced myself and asked her what the matter was.

"It is too intimate," she told me, only it came out, "Eet ees too eentemate." Now she was crying uncontrollably.

"Too intimate?" was the most intelligent reply I could come up with. Oh, God, I thought, do I really want to get into this? But I could see she was really suffering. "What is too intimate?" I asked.

"It is too embarrassing," was the answer.

"I see." Stalling for more time to determine what her concern was, and to let her get control of herself, I checked her pulse and blood pressure. They were fine. Her heart and lungs were normal.

"Do you still hear music?" I ventured.

My patient eyed me warily. "You don't?" she queried.

I recognized her accent as being similar to my grandmother's: eastern European. The kerchief too was familiar. She had probably emigrated at about the same time, I thought. My own grandmother and I had spent long hours together, drinking tea and discussing her childhood, politics, and life. The strong samovar brew drunk with cubes of white sugar and our talks warmed me. When she died a few months ago I felt as if my tie to that old world had been severed.

My patient and I shared a moment of silence, then I asked her about her origins. She seemed pleased but was guarded in her replies. She had come to talk about the present. I asked her how she spent her time.

"I paint, I listen to music, I go shopping," she said unenthusiastically.

"Family?" I asked. "Friends?"

She once again began to weep. "Old people are too boring," she said. We looked at one another.

Finally, chest heaving, she said, "It is very silly really. I am just a silly old woman." She paused and gazed at a fly that crawled across the examining table.

"He is much younger than I am," she continued. "Much younger. It is foolish. He helps me carry my groceries. He fixes things. I am sure I am just an old woman to him."

I must have been staring at her; when she turned toward me, I suddenly felt very warm and self-conscious.

She stopped weeping and looked directly at me. "But I have never felt this way about a man. I was married for 31 years, and I have never felt like this."

In the last afternoon light that filtered through the buildings surrounding the clinic, I could make out, buried in the folds of redundant skin, the features of a vital and beautiful woman, full of love and hungry for life.

"I am a silly old woman, yes?"

I looked and she was again a frail old lady, smiling sadly. I told her that love comes to all ages, that feelings cannot be right or wrong. I said other things that I could claim no right to say to a survivor of 82 years. I felt foolish.

I realized, however, that it made no difference what I said. She had been unburdened of her terrible secret. I hadn't laughed; I was not disgusted. She had found what she had come for.

I saw her again a week later. Our session was brief.

"Thank you," she said. "I was just mourning my lost youth. I realize this."

I was sorry to see her go. Feeling terribly young with much to learn, I began to examine the chart of my next patient.

By the Numbers

Nancy L. Greengold, MD

Ten! Ten!" boomed a thickly accented voice over the cacophony of the emergency room. "Ten! Ten! Ten! Ten!" The attending for the day smirked at me knowingly. "Ah, Mr R is back! The man who's always got ten-out-of-ten chest pain. So vat's new?" He turned casually to the desk clerk, ordered a stat ECG, and motioned for me to see the patient.

I first saw all the service patients—that was the resident's job. Most spoke Russian or Farsi, necessitating a translator. I marched over to Mr R, pleased to hear at least some English emanating from his mouth. "What brings you here today, Mr R?" I shouted my best open-ended question above the din of the corridor. "Ten, ten!" he replied, clutching his left breast. "Ten, ten!" Then, as if to flesh out his vocabulary, he added, "Very pain, very pain." "OK," I assured him, "so where does it hurt?" "Ten, ten!" he answered impatiently. "I know, I know. But when did it start and how long has it lasted and . . ." Mr R shook his fist at me: "Very pain! Very pain!" And then he played his final card: "Morphine!" he announced.

I walked away, frustrated with his limited fluency in English and his one-track mind. Why this preoccupation with "ten"? I pondered. I wanted to know the quality of the pain, not quantity. Clearly, Mr R had been here before, had contempt for my questions, and was cutting to the chase. "Ten!"

I paged a Farsi translator. After 15 minutes filled with the constant belching of "Ten!" from Mr R, the interpreter arrived, greeted her old friend, and extracted this history: The patient had had chest pain every day for nine months, relieved with morphine. Today he had chest pain again. And, it was ten out of ten.

The ECG was done and compared with one from the day before. No change from baseline. "Ten, ten!" shouted Mr R, noting our weary unconcern.

A commotion erupted at the adjacent bed. Whispers of "Whopping ST elevation" and "Code white" flew from beyond the curtain. The patient was English-speaking and had his attending at the bedside. "Mr J, on a scale of one to ten, how much does it hurt?" "Six," replied the diaphoretic man, "it's a six." "Call the cardiac fellow," ordered the attending. "We'll need streptokinase, stat!"

ECG notwithstanding, the number six had to be established to command full respect, it appeared. People were now running, strapping monitors on Mr J, pushing morphine and Lasix. I wondered whether a more stoic patient with a three and the same electrical vectors would be taken less seriously.

Poor Mr R couldn't figure out why he was getting short shrift. He was not receiving the attention owed a ten! Although my attending planned to admit him to the CCU for the standard rule-out, obviously there was no hurry.

I telephoned the unit resident. "I hear you guys know this man, Mr R?" Furor exploded over the line. "Know him? He's in our unit more than he's out, always with ten-out-of-ten pain. It used to buy him a bed here, but no more! All he wants is morphine!" Then the voice added, "Look, this character's clearly got some coronary artery disease, but he's refused all interventions. He won't be cathed. Last time he was in the ER we sent him home. Hold him there and we'll be down to write the discharge. You guys won't be responsible."

I ordered some morphine for Mr R, then joined my attending who was reassessing a woman with abdominal pain. He was troubled by a two-hour pain rise from five to eight. I was amazed at the power of the rating scale; it was literally tipping the balance toward considering surgery.

If quantitative claims were all-important, why then were we summarily ignoring Mr R's ten? Why didn't he get an automatic nitroglycerin drip? Had he lost credibility because of his rating-scale inflation? Would a judicious past use of fives and sixes have strengthened his current case? Mr R always got the stat ECG regardless of whether he was believed. Was our pain scale of any relevance, after all? What had we taught him, in his numerous encounters with our system, about the focus of our concerns, and more importantly, what did his language-limited attempt to gratify his desires teach us about our methods?

The attending would likely argue that the value of the pain rating scale was its relativity, enabling us to monitor the progress of symptoms. It isn't enough to record a patient's report of "worse." We need numerical validation.

I shouldn't have been surprised. Indeed, I had been taught in medical school to describe the world by the numbers. Muscle strength is 1 to 5, reflexes 0 to 4, pitting edema trace to 4+, heart murmurs 1 to 6, pulses 0 to 4.

We forego the discriminating richness of our language to embrace the homogeneity of number. Our fetal well-being is assessed not by our ample fluid or vigorous movement, but by our Biophysical Profile, 0 to 10. We descend(!) into the world from stations -3 to +3, not from high to low, and are born not limp or livid, but with Apgars 1 to 10. The New York Heart Association's claim to immortality is I to IV, I being best. Prostates enlarge, retinas deteriorate, cancers grow, by 4's. Cervical intraepithelial neoplasia runs a range of I to III, which, in turn, becomes cervical cancer stage 0 on a scale of 1 to 4. Anybody above room temperature is entitled to a Glasgow Coma Scale of at least 3. Psychiatrists inventory our depressions, 0 to 63, 63 being really bummed; neurologists mini-measure our mental statuses, 0 to 30, 30 being as sharp as the examiner. In the attempt to tabulate, compute, and graph the subjective, we use rating scales to adorn our otherwise fishy assessments with their scientific aroma.

"Ten!"

Mr R was seen by the CCU team and discharged home as promised.

At about 5 PM, I heard his familiar voice honking its way into the ER. "Ten, ten!" he announced. The emergency staff broke into pathetic laughter. "He's baa-aack!" someone clowned.

Mr R looked the same as he had, patiently clutching his breast. The new nurse on the shift was gathering vitals and ritualistically asking, "Any allergies to medicine?" "Very pain!" he seethed at her. "All right, all right, dear," she said. "On a scale of one to ten . . ." I moved away, called automatically for a stat ECG.

I couldn't believe my eyes. This time his ST segments were flying high. The T waves mocked us in their perverse inversion. The attending was stunned. The emergency room personnel sprang to action in the direction of Mr R, who looked almost elated to hear he was having an acute myocardial infarction. "Ten, ten!" he snapped at me, as if to say, "Told you so." "Ten, ten!"

Mr R was accepted graciously into the CCU that night, and died three days and two catheterizations later.

———————————

Nobody in the emergency room speaks of him anymore. But the lessons of his passage are palpable in the air. Sometimes, during a lull in the ER patient onslaught, when we've finished typing our diabetics, I and II; degreeing our burns, 1st, 2nd, and 3rd; phenotyping our hyperlipopro-teinemias, I, II, III, IV, and V; and we're ready to drift off into our own stages of sleep, 1 through 4, we remember Mr R. We remember his pidgin attempts to accommodate our quantitative analysis, and we remember our formulaic responses to his entreaties.

Very pain. (Ten.)

Laphroaig

John T. Lynn III, MD

Mrs Coolidge called to tell me about the accident. Her car, a direct descendent of the Sherman tank, was scarcely blemished; she was badly bruised and felt a little woozy. The other driver, a young woman in gym clothes, was emotionally shaken, especially after seeing how compact her Volvo had become.

Mrs Coolidge told the police officer that at the age of 95 she did not have the time to visit the emergency room. That was such expensive nonsense anyway. Tactfully—and courageously, I thought—he suggested that she put a "For Sale" sign on her windshield and leave her car in the grocery store parking lot. He drove her home and made her promise to see me.

In the humble shadow of her apartment building, my car purred to a stop. I listened to the final measures of a '60s anthem, something about a revolution. As I reached for her address on the dashboard, a plastic cup rolled over, splashing taco sauce on my beige pants. Damn it, I thought, how did she talk me into a house call?

I stalked the premises, impatiently searching for her apartment. The sweet smell of the elderly hung in the air. A familiar voice scratched its way through one of the screen windows: "Let yourself in, John."

She slouched in a Lazy-Boy chair next to a lamp that dimly lit an old picture of some middle-aged people standing on a mountain summit. She carefully took the bag of ice away from her battered right eye and grimaced. Deep forehead grooves tracked down her cheeks to her lips, forming a circle. Thin skin stretched over the purple eggs on her forearms.

"You really took a beating," I observed.

"I wish they'd left me in the gutter," she replied.

"Do you have a headache or blurry vision? Are you dizzy or weak?"

"All of the above, none of the above—does it really matter?" she snapped.

"Since you don't feel like talking, at least let me examine you."

"If you insist."

Gently, I wrapped the blood pressure cuff around her arm; then I felt for bumps and cracks under her soft white hair. Stethoscope against her chest, I lowered my head, as if in prayer, and noticed that her nylon-covered legs were muscular and full—after nearly ten decades of life.

A piece of my office stationery, taped to the wall, flapped in the breeze that entered through the screen door. It warned: "DO NOT RESUSITATE!" Between and above the "S" and the "I" a tremulous "C" had been added.

I chuckled. "I remember writing that order several years ago."

"Yes," she said, "I put it right in the doorway where the paramedics can't miss it. I even corrected your spelling so that there would be no misunderstanding of my intentions."

"Well, I think you'll be all right this time. All I can find are some scrapes and bruises."

She pointed to the kitchen counter. "Now that that's settled, why don't we have a drink?"

I grasped the bottle by the neck and mumbled, "La-fro-eeg." I recalled her Christmas gift—several finger breadths of scotch in an old peanut butter jar—and how I had mistaken the gift for a sample of concentrated urine.

"Oh, this is good stuff. Maybe I will have a nip." I paused. "But it might not be good for you to have a drink so soon after the accident."

"For goodness sakes, John, if you don't pour me one, I'll hobble over there and do it myself."

Defeated, I made the drinks, hers with extra water.

"Tell me about La-froje," I asked, stumbling over the pronunciation again.

"'La-froig' is Gaelic for 'beautiful hollow by the sea.' It's a single malt scotch made in the Hebrides, by shepherds, I suppose. They make fires with island peat to dry the malt, then age the scotch in oak casks for years, until it matures to perfection."

We sipped silently. I could taste the smoky malt, and I imagined shepherds huddled by the fire, shivering in the salty arctic wind.

"What's it like getting old, Esther?" I almost choked; calling an elderly woman by her first name went against the earliest lessons of my childhood.

"It's perfectly disgusting. My husband and friends are gone; I'm really the only one who remembers them. I'm lucky that my son is still here. He's getting on too, you know. This year I retired from the Chorale. They wanted me to stay, of course, but I kept imagining whispers in the audience, 'Who's the frog in the front row?' And now I'll give up driving and have to rely on my young friends. Aging strips away the pleasures and necessities of life one by one."

"Did you ever," I interrupted, "read that Henry James story in which the old Englishman refused to have his portrait painted until his 90th birthday? He waited until the whole man, experienced and wise, would be there on the canvas to guide future generations of the family."

"By the time a person's 90, there isn't much left to paint," she scowled.

"Well, I don't think I'll convince you of whatever I'm trying to say. Just remember that you mean a lot to many people in this town, and to me," I said.

"I like you," she said. "Bedside manner has always been more important to me than clinical competence."

Heat radiated from my cheeks. "I accept the compliment . . . I think." We laughed.

"You see," she said, "at my age it's difficult even to deliver a compliment properly."

"Call me if you are not feeling better soon, will you?"

She nodded. Her left eye was moist.

A shadow covered my car while pink clouds watched the sun, exhausted, drop behind Pikes Peak. I found a Bach prelude on the radio and drove home on the back streets.

Babu

Mark S. Smith, MD

He was old and grizzled and lay under a blanket on his cot in the corner of the men's section of Mother Teresa's House for the Destitute and Dying at Kalighat. He hardly made a sound as we worked to clean his wounds, probing and pulling out the maggots that had infested his nose and gums. His nose was completely eroded in several places, across the bridge and over the nostrils. Inside his mouth the upper gums were lacerated, leaving large channels opening directly into his nasal cavity. It was not clear what the primary problem had been (cancer? trauma? infection?), but now he was in extremis and the maggots were writhing in all of these cavities. The staff, a German volunteer and two Bengalis, thought the maggots had eaten away his face and had been removing them carefully for several days. I suggested that they were just debriding necrotic tissue, but the staff persisted in their belief in the primary role of maggots in the destruction of normal tissue. I kept silent. It really didn't matter now, since good nursing care and removal of the maggots—whatever their action—seemed appropriate. I held an old, battery-operated lantern, with my thumb carefully keeping the glass and reflector from falling off, and illuminated the field as they removed the maggots with forceps. A Bengali worker everted a nostril or the upper lip as we searched the fleshy cavities that had once been intact tissue, looking for the elusive quarter-inch maggots as they hid like moray eels in a sea cave. Applying ether locally brought them wriggling out of their burrows, where they could be grasped and removed. For more than half an hour we extracted about 30 of these small creatures as the old man stoically lay still and only occasionally moaned as we tugged at pieces of loose tissue mistaken for maggots. "Babu, Babu," said the German in soft, reassuring tones followed by Bengali phrases that must have been of encouragement and care. Then, in English, as he extracted maggot after maggot, he muttered, "Such suffering, such suffering."

Jailhouse Blues

Joseph E. Paris, MD

The clanking ritual proceeds smoothly as I am once again identified and then nodded through the nine motorized steel gates. When I first made the trek through the Florida State Prison Clinic, I felt uneasy about those thick iron bars. Now that I am a three-year veteran of several state prisons, my only reaction to the slow-opening gates is one of impatience.

I never got used to my monthly trip to the high-security prison. I'm more comfortable with my hospital appointment at the lower-security prison nearby, where the staff of 12 other physicians makes being a prison doctor more tolerable. Even there the question returns: Is this what I went to medical school for?

I stopped looking for the answer a long time ago, and even my wife has come to terms with my spending much of my day behind bars: I have never been physically threatened by a prisoner.

The contrast between the medieval prison buildings and the comparatively modern hospital at the prison medical center is even more noticeable today. The old, musty fortress is being painted one more time, and the just-sanded walls reveal scores of paint layers, much like an archeological excavation site. Everything matches: the examination room has been primed with gray, the day is gray, and I will soon see inmates whose sentences are sometimes measured in centuries. Even the town's name is oddly appropriate: Starke, Florida.

My patient is a curious amalgam of youth and decay. The deterioration—so common in inmates—is manifested in his missing teeth, slumped shoulders, distinctive scars, and receding hairline. But his sparkling eyes—too blue to be old—betray his real age of 23. Like the seven patients who preceded him, he has been brought to me in handcuffs and leg shackles. I motion the guard to remove them, as I always do.

What crime was he convicted of? It's never found in the medical chart, and I make a point not to ask the security officers. Knowing may taint my medical judgment. But I can't help wondering if he committed murder, rape, or some other serious crime, like most of the inmates. To me, he is another patient-prisoner to be processed. Yet I find myself trying to establish a human contact, a frame of reference. No such luck. His physical demeanor and thick chart are so average that his name could very well be Joe Prisoner.

The consultation request contains a familiar statement: "Please see this white male with unexplained weight loss and lymphadenopathy." I begin my routine examination automatically, while my mind wanders ahead, mapping his future.

He will soon enter the prison hospital. After I counsel him and obtain his consent, he will undergo serum HIV antibody determinations and T-cell profiles, x-rays, lymph node biopsies, possibly a bronchoscopy and other tests. He will see some of the other unfortunate men in various stages of the disease. He will cling to a last ray of hope: "Is there any chance that your tests are wrong, Doctor?"

Sooner or later, if he is lucky enough to survive his first opportunistic infection, he will be assigned a bed in the AIDS Unit. He will share his few remaining years of life with a couple dozen inmates with the disease who wile away their time watching TV and bickering with the medical personnel, the security officers, and each other. I will be this man's primary physician and the likely target of much of his anger. He will ask, "Why me? I know scads of guys who shot drugs, slept with prostitutes, had homosexual experiences! Why me?"

Why him indeed? How did he get AIDS? Does it matter now?

My daydreams of this man's future blur as I envision his stays at and discharges from the AIDS Unit, each time a little weaker. There will be one last, lengthy stay culminating with the ultimate complication: death, which will restore simplicity.

My reverie is interrupted as I realize he has spoken for the first time. "Well, Doc, what do you think?" I look at him, knowing what is in store, wishing I didn't. He observes me carefully. He knows I know. We make eye contact for the first time. In a flash, somehow, he knows too. The whites of his eyes turn pink as he slumps back, overwhelmed. I try to reassure him that no diagnosis can be made until I receive the reports of the tests. My voice sounds hollow, but I can't afford to get involved. There is too much to be done, for him and for the others.

In *One Day in the Life of Ivan Denisovitch,* Siberian prisoner Ivan wonders: "How can a man who is warm understand a man who is cold?" I feel a little like Ivan's guard: How can a man without AIDS understand the plight of a man with AIDS? To be able to care for this man, however, I must withdraw, to protect myself and my own drained emotions. I rise quickly and summon the security officer. "Next patient, please."

The Last Death Song

Steven F. Gordon, MD

Death came as no surprise to Mary. She lay in her bed and sang. The third floor of the deteriorating Indian Hospital rang with her voice.

She was very old. When Mary had been born, the Battle of Wounded Knee was still news, and the Bureau of Indian Affairs' policy encouraged the sale of reservation lands to non-Indians. The memories of the tribe's five forced moves in 30 years were as strong in her society's memory as the memory of the Holocaust is today. The peyote church came to the reservation and replaced the warrior societies as the social organizing force when Mary was mastering literacy of her own language. The clan system was deteriorating at the beginning of World War II when her grandchildren started to arrive. English had replaced Hochungra as the reservation's main language at the end of the war, and by that time written Hochungra had been abandoned. Mary was already considered old in the 1950s, when penicillin became readily available and the Indian Health Service was removed from the Bureau of Indian Affairs and put under the auspices of the Public Health Service. She had to wait until close to the age of 70 to be granted full religious freedom by the Supreme Court, and she was 80 when the tribal government started buying back the land that had been sold when she was a child. She was 90 when the reservation hospital ceased being a referral center for the Indian Health Service. She was close to a century old when I came to the reservation and she sang her death song.

I took the history from her family because Mary wouldn't (and couldn't) talk to me. We stood in the hallway (there was no family conference room), and I leaned against the peeling-paint walls and took notes.

A robust, heterogeneous group, my informants spanned several generations. Their accents ranged from soft lilting to flat Midwestern. Mary kept singing as we talked.

For as long as anyone in the family or on the reservation could remember, Mary had been in good health. Three days before coming to the hospital, she began to cough and had run a high fever. She had refused hospitalization, but as her condition worsened she was unable to refuse any longer, and her relatives brought her in.

As I walked into Mary's room, her singing filled my mind. Her frail, not quite 80-pound body was an incongruous sight below the cavernous 1930s-vintage ceiling. Her pure white hair accentuated her facial pallor in the dingy light. Her eyes were sunken and her cheeks hollow. Her bony hands were tightly crossed over her chest as she sang with her eyes closed. She didn't stop singing during my exam, nor did she even seem aware I was there.

Her blood pressure was undetectable, her pulse weak and thready. The skin on the backs of her hands "tented" up but did not go down. Rales filled her chest. Her fingers and toes were blue.

Her lab work was less than encouraging: high creatinine, low WBC count, profound anemia, low sodium, elevated liver function values.

Clearly, Mary's septic shock, pulmonary edema, dehydration, and renal failure required a more sophisticated medical facility. Our lab couldn't do blood gases. The closest thing to an ICU was a small, empty room attached to the nurses' station. We had no cardiac monitor, continuous blood pressure monitoring, or staff who could handle a dopamine drip.

Her family surrounded me as I walked back into the hall. Although Mary's prognosis was poor, I recommended transfer off the reservation to the nearest full-service hospital, 25 miles away.

Her family refused. They didn't want respirators, dialysis, or ICUs. If death was near, they wished Mary to die close to home and family.

It was my first encounter with the Hochungra belief that matters of life and death are best left in the hands of the Author of life and death.

Mary was ready for death and she sang.

Death songs were a tradition among many Plains tribes, particularly among those who spoke Siouan languages, such as the Dakota, Osage, Crow, and Hochungra. I had read about death songs some years before, but had thought they had vanished with the warrior tradition. I certainly had never expected to hear one.

The songs themselves were highly individualized; their purpose was to prepare the singer both spiritually and psychologically for death. Mary's song seemed to be one phrase of Hochungra, repeated four times, followed by one phrase of English, also repeated four times.

With Mary's relatives now gathered around her, I administered "ordinary medical care": IV fluids and antibiotics. She tenaciously sang her death song throughout that day, until my shift ended. The next morning she was still singing, and she sang into the next night, when I was on call. She sang well into the afternoon. By the morning of the third hospital day, she had stopped singing.

Incredibly, she recovered and was soon discharged to a nursing home.

The place was 30 miles from the reservation in a non-Indian farming community. Among the few Indians there were two elderly Hochungra women whom I visited every month or so. I visited Mary too, but she invariably complained about the place. I learned that her relatives visited her frequently and took her on outings, but she never spoke of it to me. I never saw her smile.

Like so many "government doctors" before me, I eventually left the Indian Health Service, pushed by shattered idealism and bureaucratic frustrations, and pulled by better money elsewhere. A year later I learned that Mary had died.

I pondered her death and began to wonder if I had done either the patient or her community a service by snatching her from sure death. She had been ready to die, her family and her community had been ready for her death. My therapy had shattered the integrity of her final life event.

I have since asked myself many times: Did she sing her death song again? Did anyone know what she was singing? Had I heard the last death song?

Flaky

Ronald A. Katz, MD

It was a beautiful, warm afternoon in September when I first met Daniel. He stood rather apprehensively in the center of the examination room, dressed, it seemed, for winter. On a day when I had already seen several other students dressed in T-shirts and shorts, Daniel wore a long-sleeved flannel shirt buttoned to the neck and baggy corduroy slacks. His large, sad eyes were almost hidden by his hair, which was carefully combed down over his forehead, giving him the appearance of someone who might have been just released after being institutionalized for many years. In fact, he was a new college freshman in the school of engineering at the state university near my office, and had been referred to me by the student health service.

"Doc," he blurted, "I can't stand it anymore. I just want to be able to be with other people without having them look at me like I'm a leper, like they might catch what I have. I want to be able to hold a girl's hand, to go to the beach in the summer. Please. Please help me." As he began to undress, fine silvery scales fell freely in a shower around him. I was reminded of the forlorn snowman in a fluid-filled paperweight that would "snow" only when agitated. As I looked at the large, thick plaques of psoriasis covering most of his body, I could only begin to imagine the effect this disease had already had on his life.

Gradually and haltingly, over many months, Daniel told me his story. He had grown up in a small town in the economically depressed western part of the state. He had had a streptococcal pharyngitis when he was 10, which was treated appropriately with penicillin by his family physician. As his sore throat improved, however, a generalized rash began to develop, characterized by tiny, red, scaly lesions shaped like teardrops. These "guttate" lesions continued to grow into larger papules and plaques, coalescing in some areas, eventually covering three fourths of his body. Then, lesions appeared on his face and scalp, making it impossible for him to completely conceal his disease.

Attempts at camouflage caused him to don inappropriate clothing and to style his hair in such a peculiar way. Even worse, he told me months later, if he sat or stood in one place for more than a few minutes, a puddle of silvery white scales collected at his feet, making him the unhappy recipient of a cruel nickname, Flaky, bestowed on him by thoughtless classmates. Daniel wept as he told me this story of the name that had stayed with him until he finally left home for college.

His family physician had done what he could, providing free care and samples of topical corticosteroids, but the psoriasis was too severe to respond to this minimal therapy, and Dan's family was too poor to travel elsewhere for specialized care. He soon discovered that the sun helped his disease, but he continued to cover up even on the hottest summer days because of embarrassment and self-consciousness.

In fact, his efforts to hide his disease became a pervasive obsession throughout his childhood and adolescence. His nervous anticipation of unabashed stares and crude remarks created his life-style of protective behavior. He never dated, or went swimming, or took up a sport, which he was sure would draw jeers from the other students. He had few friends, spending almost all his free time studying in hopes he might earn a scholarship that would take him away from the place where he had suffered so much shame.

Once Daniel reached the university, he was determined to get help. But first he secured a part-time job so he would be able to pay something toward his treatment. Soon after our first meeting he started photochemotherapy (PUVA: oral psoralen plus long-wavelength ultraviolet light). Within eight weeks his skin was 75% clear of the disease that had devastated his life for eight years. Did this dramatically change his life? You bet it did!

As his outward appearance improved, so did his self-image. His dress, facial expressions, and general social interactions began to reflect his new confidence and his new life. Was he cured? Of course not. But as our relationship matured, he realized his disease could be controlled. That relationship—developed over many years—was based on more than my simply prescribing drugs to stop the progression of his disease. He learned that stress played an important role in flareups, as did other minor physical illnesses. For that reason, he needed to know I was there to share all aspects of his life. Regular visits, even when his skin was well controlled, allowed us to continually renew that initial bond, which seemed to give him the confidence he needed to continue his battle.

Daniel has remained my patient for ten years. He is a nice-looking young man with a wife, children, and a successful career. His disease will always be part of his life, but it no longer dominates it. Because of him I have learned that treating severe psoriasis—or any disfiguring condition—requires more than just implementing the latest drug therapy. Daniel needed someone he could trust, someone who wasn't repelled by his physical appearance. He needed someone who really understood his misery, and who shared his success.

John Updike[1] eloquently compared this life-long struggle with psoriasis to life as a leper:

> Each morning, I vacuum my bed. My torture is skin deep: there is no pain, not even itching; we lepers live a long time, and are ironically healthy in other respects. Lusty, though we are loathsome to love. Keen-sighted, though we hate to look upon ourselves. The name of the disease, spiritually speaking, is Humiliation.

1. Updike J. From the journal of a leper. *The New Yorker.* July 19, 1976:28-33.

The Man Who Didn't Know He Had Cancer

Adria Burrows, MD

When I was called by the internist for an ophthalmology consultation, he mentioned something I thought rather odd.

"Mr Martin doesn't know he's dying of cancer," he said. "It was his family's wish, and I abided by it. He thinks he has a bad virus, so don't say anything." It seemed strange to me and yet it was possible. What would I have done as the internist? Could I keep such a "secret"? As the consultant, however, luckily I didn't have to make that decision.

Mr Martin was a thin, delicate-looking man who was propped up on three pillows when I came to see him. Pictures of his family filled an end table and a thick novel lay on his lap. He had been in the hospital for a while. He held out his hand and shook mine with surprising strength for someone so cachectic.

"So, you're the ophthalmologist," he said with a grin. "Probably the only doctor in the hospital I haven't met yet." I nodded and asked what kind of problem he was having. "My vision is very blurry in the morning when I wake up. It gets better as the day goes on. Like now, it's normal."

That was a disturbing symptom in someone with cancer, as it usually means there is papilledema from brain metastases.

Mr Martin's vision was indeed perfect when I saw him, but as I examined the backs of his eyes with my ophthalmoscope, the swollen optic nerves glared back at me.

"So, what is it, Doc?"

"Swollen nerves," I answered.

"From what?"

"We'll need a CT scan to know."

Mr Martin nodded. "Is it from the virus?" he asked.

"Could be." I felt uncomfortable but told him I would keep him posted.

"All the doctors say that. You think they mean it?"

"I do." I shook his hand again and left.

Mr Martin's scan did show multiple metastases in the brain. How aggressive would his physicians be? Would they tell him that the radiation they wanted to give him was for a virus? Would he continue to believe them?

The next time I was on Mr Martin's floor, it was to write preop notes on another patient early one morning. As I sat at the dim, deserted nurses' station, I saw Willie approaching. Willie, an orderly, was always cheerful and bright-eyed. I waved to him. I had done cataract surgery on both Willie and his wife, and ever since, Willie and I had often shared opinions about patients: mine, from the physician's point of view, and Willie's, from talking with patients as he transported them. Willie had a talent for opening up to people, and thus the frightened or nervous patient on a stretcher or in a wheelchair felt comfortable sharing his or her feelings.

"How's it going?" Willie asked.

"Fine."

"Who you writing on?"

"Henderson."

"Henderson. At least she knows what's going on. Got a great family. Not like Martin's."

"What about Martin?"

"You saw him. You know the story. His family don't want him to know nothing. Every time his wife comes to visit, she tells him he'll go home next week. Just got to fight off that virus. Been telling him for a month now and each day he gets weaker and weaker. He's not leaving so soon and she knows it. He's not stupid, though. He knows everything."

"You mean he knows?" I asked. Willie nodded.

"I was in his room really early one day, picking him up for a bone scan. Came with a wheelchair, and he sighed really heavy and said he don't want to go. 'What's the use?' he said. 'I'm going to die and I know it.' I told him he is not and he got extra mad and told me to stop lying. 'I get lies from my family, my wife . . . I don't need more from you. We might as well be honest with each other. I got liver cancer and that's that.' So, he told me everything and now we talk a lot. I even go to see him before I go home sometimes, and we talk about his illness, his family, and stuff. He's a good guy and he's just playing along with the game."

"Why doesn't he tell his wife or doctor that he knows?" I asked.

"Why should he? Then, he said, everyone will act even stranger than they do now. They'll cry and mourn, and he don't need to see that." Willie saluted me and began to walk away. "Don't you be telling anyone what I just said." He turned a corner and disappeared.

What would I do in Mr Martin's situation? Again I was reminded of my discomfort at being a part of this deception. I started to walk to the operating room and stopped by Mr Martin's doorway as I pondered the situation. The room was dark and I could see the outline of his figure on the bed.

"Doctor?" I walked in and sat on the edge of his bed. "I want you to know something, Doc." He paused. "Before I got sick, I was the founder and owner of a big company. I needed all my wits about me all the time . . . it's competitive out there," he said, pointing to the window. "I had to know who to hire, who to fire. I could take one look at someone and tell if he's a good worker or a bum. I could tell if someone was lying or telling the truth. Being flat on your back in a hospital bed makes people think you're dumb. If you're debilitated, then you're dumb. These eyes see a lot and know a lot." I nodded.

"You heard Willie and me talking about you?"

"A little. No matter, though. I know I don't have a virus. Known that for a long time. Even without seeing the lies in my wife's eyes and my doctor's face, I can tell my body is dying. A flu doesn't make you this thin. A flu doesn't make your doctor order brain scans, bone scans, and medicine that makes you vomit. You see, we always know what's going on. You're a young doctor and I hope you learn a lesson from me. Be honest with your patients. Tell the family it's not healthy to keep secrets. It just weaves a web of confusion and deception." He smiled. "I went bankrupt once, years ago. Didn't want to tell my wife. I just told her no more allowance and no more steak. You can't fool her . . . the minute I came home with my sad face, she knew something was up. I told her I just wanted to save up for this boat cruiser I had my eye on, but she knew. In fact, *she* told *me* we were bankrupt even without seeing the books, just based on reading my eyes. She knew then and I know now. She thinks I can't read her face, but I can."

"Why don't you tell her?"

"I can't, Doc. I don't want to talk to her about illness or death. I like when she comes, brings me a hamburger I can't eat, tells me about her day, how she's preparing the house for my return, a welcome-home party. I'd rather hear about that and pretend it's really going to happen. I know where I'm going from here: the hospice. Ah, don't look like that, Doc. I face up to my problems. Always did. Willie and I talk a lot, too . . . he's like my therapist."

I shook Mr Martin's hand. "You're a brave man," I said.

"Bravery is in the eyes of the beholder. Now just remember what I said and get going. You have better things to do than listen to an old man. And I want to sleep."

I stood, patted him on the shoulder, and left. I was glad I had had the chance to talk with him openly and pleased too that he could confide in Willie. I realized that somehow I'd been "spoiled" as an ophthalmologist, telling patients all day long and quite matter-of-factly whether they had glaucoma or cataracts or healthy eyes. There were never any secrets in my examining room. Then again, I don't deal with life-and-death situations. Perhaps if I did, I might fall into charades such as this. No. I doubted it. It bothered me to hold honesty back when confronting illness. Why should I or a patient feel uncomfortable? Why should we not be able to share everything?

My name was paged and I knew my operating room was ready. I quickened my step and caught the elevator. There were no longer any secrets weighing on my mind.

A Purely Cosmetic Procedure

Alan Rockoff, MD

W hy on earth would you *want* to remove tattoos?"

When my colleagues discover that I remove tattoos in my practice, they are puzzled and skeptical. What motive could a physician have for doing that sort of thing, other than the obvious one, greed? Bad enough to use lasers (or other means) to rid patients of birthmarks or scars or other defects. We dismiss such concerns as "cosmetic," which is to say trivial and frivolous. In the medical construction of reality, a cosmetic problem is not "real," not something physicians consider important enough to fix, diagnose, or at least define in conventional terms. Insurers seem to validate this construction in the most potent way possible: by reimbursing only for those problems physicians count as real.

Foolish enough, then, to bother with marks that, however petty, are at least acts of nature. But tattoos? Do people who deform themselves deserve anyone's interest or skill to undo the predictable results of their own folly?

Some of my colleagues' questions sound faint but clear class under-tones. As one put it, lowering his voice a bit (although we were alone), "Do you really want the kind of clientele that has tattoos?" That clientele is plainly not "our sort" of people. Who are these tattoo types, anyway? What motivates them? What are they after? Why do they mutilate them-selves in the first place, and how will they react if treatment doesn't pro-duce the results they expect? One never knows about these "cosmetic sorts." They may be unrealistic. Their very concerns mark them as neurotic and unhappy with themselves.

I was about 15, I guess. I grew up on the east side of town, the poorer side. Nobody paid much attention to what I was doing, so I was out on the streets by the time I was in ninth grade. You know—broken home, alcoholic father, Mom too busy trying to keep the house going to pay much attention to my sisters or me.

I don't remember exactly how it happened. Just one night a bunch of us got together and drove to a town downstate. One of my buddies said he knew a guy who had a tattoo parlor there, and we all had one put on. It didn't hurt too much. I remember the tattoo guy gave me a choice of designs. This tattoo he put here on my arm—I don't even think it's the one I picked, but it didn't matter, as long as I had one. You can see it when I wear a short-sleeved shirt.

My in-laws have been very nice. Really, they never mention it at all, but my father-in-law did say he would pay for it if I wanted it off. He's a big attorney downtown, and he's on the board of trustees at the university. My wife grew up a lot different from the way I did. Like I said, I'm from the other side of the tracks and she's from the good part of town, where her folks still live. They have some house, you should see it. They give parties there all the time, for the attorneys in her dad's firm and for the trustees at the university. And like I said, her family's awfully nice. They've always accepted me, ever since my wife brought me home to meet them.

And now I have a house of my own! It's small, two bedrooms. My wife and I use one, and the girls are in the other; one's 3 and the other's 6 months. I started my own business last year. It's going pretty well, but I still do some work for my old boss to help make the house payments. Between the two jobs, we'll be OK.

I look at myself and I can hardly believe it. Here I am, 32 years old, with a wife, two kids, a house, and my own business. I don't even recognize myself. When I was 15, I never pictured myself doing any of these things. I can't even really figure out how it all happened.

This tattoo on my arm, I guess it was a stupid thing to do, a kid thing. Whenever I look at it, it reminds me of who I was then. My wife and my in-laws look at it too, but like I said, they're too nice to say anything.

And then I look at who I am now. This tattoo reminds me where I came from. But I'm not the kind of person who would put a tattoo on, at least not anymore. And you know, sometimes I think maybe it isn't right for me to be taking it off like this. Maybe I don't deserve to forget where I come from.

During this soliloquy the laser beats out a steady tattoo of its own, with a fluence of seven joules per square centimeter. Each second a pulse of light, wavelength 755 nanometers, carves another three-millimeter disk out of the young man's unwanted tattoo. Seventeen years ago, in a group ritual with ancient roots and complex, unfathomable meanings, he had his class and social origins inscribed in his flesh. Now, crafting a new identity, he is having the brand expunged. The completed process will leave no scar, at least none anyone else can see.

His concerns, it goes without saying, are purely cosmetic. That is to say, they are airy and insubstantial, too trivial to engage the notice or warrant the attention of any self-respecting member of the healing profession.

The Hymn

David N. Little, MD

As I made rounds at the nursing home, accompanied by the charge nurse, occasional shrill cries echoed in the corridors. We stopped in a room to check on one of our patients, and the ambient sounds continued at a slightly muffled level. I thought to myself that the slight woman in the wheelchair probably could not hear most of the background noise. She could hardly see who might have come to visit. One eye was closed and oozing from a chronic infection. The lens had been replaced in the other eye, but she seemed to have difficulty focusing on our faces. I could not be sure if the lack of eye contact was due to the blankness of cognitive impairment or simply to the decline in her visual acuity. Yet there was something dignified about her, the neat beige skirt and lacy white blouse rumpled only by the folds of the wheelchair cushion. I wanted to know her better.

The nurse knew how to get her attention, avoiding direct eye contact in favor of a gentle touch and reassuring voice. "The doctor is here to see you."

"Well, I wish I could see him," came the wistful reply, "and I wish he could get me back home." She seemed resigned to her circumstances, but there was just a trace of hope in her voice.

She had come to the nursing home two months ago after a fall in her apartment resulted in a fracture of the odontoid process of the second cervical vertebra. Although she had suffered no permanent neurological deficit, the initial immobilization left her weakened and unable to stand. Added to her chronic heart disease, mild memory loss, and deficits of vision and hearing, this handicap had been the straw that broke the back of her independent spirit. Her family and the hospital discharge planners judged it unsafe for her to live on her own, so she was placed in the nursing facility, 300 miles from the place she called home.

We talked about her joint pain and mobility problems, which did not seem to be improving.

"I don't think anyone can ever fix me up enough so that I can go home," said the old woman, then lapsed into her usual quiet mood.

I sensed her helplessness and despair and longed to offer some encouragement.

She had been a minister's wife and together they served in Baptist churches. With her love and talent for music, she often assumed the role of organist. These facts had surfaced briefly during her intake history at the nursing home, then took a back seat to the seemingly more urgent needs of her initial care.

Remembering this history and hoping to cheer her up, I asked about her reported interest in music. An averted head was the only response. The nurse, who had overheard my question, said there was a piano in the day room. Perhaps they might try it.

About an hour later, while sitting at the nurses' station writing progress notes, I heard faint, rather pleasant sounds and walked down the hall to investigate. I stopped at the day room, where the nurse sat on the piano bench next to the woman, gently encouraging her to play.

"Can you use your left hand too? Can you play the bass?"

For a moment, seemingly random notes came from the thin, frail fingers, but gradually a familiar hymn emerged. A slight smile appeared on the weathered face and she sang softly:

"What a friend we have in Jesus."

Monday Morning Clinic

Abigail Zuger, MD

Mr Lopez? Mr Lopez. Have a seat. Let's see the arm. Oh dear. Are you taking those pills? Are you sure? How many do you have left? How can you have a lot left? I gave you 60. You're supposed to take them four times a day. I saw you two weeks ago. So? That's what I thought. What were you saving them for? This is the rainy day, right here. Now. That's why it still hurts. It still hurts, right? I bet it does. Do you have a bathtub at home? I want you to soak it in a bathtub. Does your mother have a bathtub? Then soak it in your mother's bathtub. Twice a day. And take the antibiotics. Yours and mine. Nobody else's. More? Didn't you just say you have a lot left? I want you to take them. Not collect them. Swallow them. Well, maybe she'll let you in if you tell her you have to use her bathtub. Tell her you're sorry. Tell her your doctor said she should let you in. Tell her to call me. Oh, now, it's all right. Take it easy. No, this isn't the end. No, you're not going to croak. You just have an infection in your arm. This one has nothing to do with the virus. You just need antibiotics. And a bathtub. That's why I want to talk to her. Just about the tub. And get your blood tests done, please. See you next week.

Mr Lamb? Mr Lamb. Have a seat. Oh dear. I'll hang up your coat. A whole week like this? Why didn't you call? A hundred point five? A hundred and five. Can you breathe for me, please? Through your mouth. And again. Did you have your x-ray done? Let's take a look. Well, we seem to have a bit of a problem here. I'm sure you know what I'm going to say. I know you don't want to come in. Yes, I remember vividly what you said last time, but it really would be the best. Wait, now, just hold on. Don't leave. Take it easy. Let's try to figure something out. There's a combination of pills that sometimes works as well as the intravenous. I suppose we can try them. Sometimes, though, they can make you sick. I know you're sick. I mean sicker. Then you really will have to come in. But we can try them. What do you think? Yes, I hope so too. I want to see you here three times this week. With blood tests. If you feel worse, go to Emergency immediately. Tell them to call me. You know the routine. Is your mother outside? Home calling who? All of them? Flying in? Oh, really, I think that's extremely premature. No, not at all. Of course I would tell you. But I really don't think so. You remember, she did this the last time too. And here you are, right? Right. Now, don't worry. Of course she can call me. This one is one a day and this one is two four times a day. And blood tests. Yes, you have some blood left. I happen to know, you have some left. Well, let them try, and if they can't find a vein you can come back to me. Don't worry.

Miss Caballero? Ana, come in. You look wonderful. How are you? Nothing since Friday? Nothing at all? Why not? Well, who knows if you don't know? Are you sick? Did you have a reaction to the treatment? So why aren't you eating? Is it the end of the month—have you run out of stamps? No? Are you sure? You can tell me, you know. Sometimes we can help. You're sure? All right, let me tell you a few things. Your blood tests are almost normal now. You can stop taking the iron. You really couldn't be doing any better. How long has it been now, a year? That's fantastic. You know, that fungus is almost gone from your brain now, with those treatments. We couldn't hope for things to be better. I happen to know that everyone in that waiting room would pay money for your blood counts. Of course I mean it. No, I told you, I can't promise that. But hopefully for a long time. Well, I'm glad it does. Maybe now you'll eat a little. You were starting to worry again, weren't you? Can you come by next week? Start with soup. Don't forget your blood tests. Yes, you have enough. I happen to know, you have enough.

Mr Santos? Mr Santos, where are you? Mr Santos? Well for heaven's sake. I didn't recognize you. Sixteen pounds? Well for heaven's sake. Have a seat. It's working, then. No, not surprised, exactly, not surprised. I told you, for some people it works like a miracle. Really, to Macy's? Out all afternoon? Well. Now look, I guess we shouldn't forget that this may not last. Sometimes the virus gets used to this one too. And it has side effects. So you have to be prepared. We have to be prepared. But even so, I'm so glad. Oh, you shouldn't have done that. It's beautiful. Well, thank you. I don't know what to say. Yes, I'll bet she's happy. Will you get your blood drawn today, please? Very funny. You know you have enough. And thank Mrs Santos for me too.

Mrs Nunez? Mrs Nunez. Oh hello, como esta? One second. Too fast for me. Mr Santos, are you in a big hurry? Could you give me a hand for a second? You remember Mrs Nunez. Ah, now she recognizes you. Well. Ask her how she is. Still the same? Is it any better at all? Is she still dizzy? No, well, that's good. Listen, tell her that the test showed that she does have an infection in her bowels. A strong infection. Fuerte. Yes, I bet she knows. Tell her that I'm afraid there are no good antibiotics for this particular infection. Sometimes, though, it goes away by itself. That's what we have to hope for. What does she say? No, she shouldn't take that anymore. I'm going to give her pills that are a little stronger. I hope they help a little. Well. Ask her why she didn't bring her little girls today. Oh no, I'm sorry, now don't cry. No, now, you know it's the best thing. When you get better, maybe they can come back for a while. Does she remember, we arranged all that with the lawyer last month? Yes, come in. Oh, of course, her mother, of course I remember. Well, I suppose there's room somewhere. Here, sit over here and I'll stand. Yes, she's a little sick. I hope it will be better. No, no. Not yet. I don't think so. I hope not. Now, look, today she's better. Don't you think so? Better. We'll try hard. If the pills don't help we'll try something else. I think she should see the social worker today. And blood tests today. Funny, I understood that perfectly. Of course she has enough blood. I happen to know, she has enough. Trust me. And don't worry. Yes, who is it? Oh, Mr Atwood. It'll be just a little bit longer, I'm afraid. Yes, I know, Mr Atwood, and I'm very sorry, but you know we go in order here. Mr Atwood, as you can see, you cannot fit into this room at the moment. Please go back and have a seat outside. Here are the blood tests, Mrs Nunez, and here is the prescription. The social worker is that lady with gray hair. I'll tell her you need her. I want you back next week. Una semana, OK? Gracias. Thanks, Mr Santos.

Mr Atwood? All right, Mr Atwood, you can come back. Have a seat. Well, I'm sorry you feel that way. We certainly try not to give people the runaround here. We do the best we can. So. How are you doing? Are you still drinking? Oh, I just had a feeling. Maybe we'll just leave the door open a crack here. Yes, I got those results back on Friday. I'm afraid they've gone down a little. No, just a little. No, I know it sounds like a lot, but from 280 to 235 is really not a great deal. Well, it's possible that drinking could make them go down a little. But you remember what I explained to you about the virus bursting up your cells? Well, I think that's probably what's happening. That's why I really do think you should start taking that medicine. Yes, I suppose the drinking could be making things worse. Well, exactly how much is that? Only when you come to clinic? I know how you feel. Yes, I think you should stop too. Definitely. I know it's hard. But the problem is, Mr Atwood, that what I told you about the virus just isn't going to change. You really should be taking that medicine. I know you feel fine. But remember, we want to keep you feeling fine. Just keep thinking about it. Oh, now it's all right, none of us takes it personally. We know what a long wait in the waiting room is like. Of course you don't have to keep coming back, Mr Atwood, but I really do think it would be a good idea. You could just give the medicine a try, you know. Just for a week, and see how it goes. Sometimes it's easier if you don't think "forever." Just think a week at a time. I'll tell you what. I'll give you a prescription for two weeks. No more. Just in case you change your mind. Come see me in two weeks. Yes, I know it's hard. It's the hardest thing in the world.

Chorea

Ronald H. Lands, MD

Limited only by a soft wrist restraint, the gnarled hand moved in a repetitive, graceful motion. The fingers curved, then clasped gently to the palm with the thumb extended. The arm then tugged upward, gently, at the band anchored to the rail of the hospital bed, as if testing it. The hand rested, occasionally, on the sheets but after a time, and without obvious provocation, it worked through the same monotonous pattern again.

A diagnosis of cryptococcal meningitis explained her delirium and warranted sedation. An endotracheal tube sustained life but precluded speech. The left hand, shackled by the pain of an arterial line, remained motionless.

Our neurologist could not identify a lesion to explain such a peculiar movement. My patient, followed by her ventilator, several monitors, assorted pumps, and the nurse in command of it all, convoyed to the radiology suite where she endured a CT scan of her brain. The right hand moved rhythmically, but sporadically, several times during the procedure. The scan was of excellent quality, and a full-page typewritten report documented it to be normal.

The hand motions persisted. The action occurred with no apparent direction from the elderly head attached to the wizened body. There were no desperate searching movements of the eyes in an attempt to communicate over the barriers created by the life-support machine. The movement just repeated itself day and night, with visitors or without, on good days and bad.

A nurse on the night shift claimed she recognized the movement as a request for ICE in the language of the deaf. I was not aware that my patient had experience with the deaf or their language. Ice chips on her lips, however, seemed to cause the motions to cease for long periods of time. Even though she signed no other requests, it seemed the best answer. No one challenged it.

The reputation of the astute nurse justifiably escalated as the news of this diagnosis spread. Moral proclamations abounded. Biases were reaffirmed.

"Technology is not always the answer," the nurses said. "We must tend to the whole patient because the archaic medical model fails them." I blushed; I considered myself a progressive thinker.

"I must pay more attention to the physical examination. Those findings did not fit a specific anatomic lesion, and I, of all people, should have known better," said the neurologist in a humbled voice. My shoulders sagged with his; I considered myself a diagnostician.

"Unnecessary radiographic procedures contribute to the inflationary spiral of health care costs," said the radiologist. "A CT scan is too often normal under these circumstances. An MRI, however, might have provided some useful information," he continued. I flinched at this pronouncement; I try to be a cost-effective physician.

I, the internist, the one person expected to make a diagnosis by the powers of history and observation, did not know this singular piece of information about a patient I had treated for more than two years. While dealing with the agony of her malignancy and the toxicity of chemotherapy, she must have communicated with someone, possibly a family member, by means of sign language. I had missed this vital piece of social history. I felt unfit to wear my white clinician's coat. I resolved to do better.

She recovered slowly. Sequentially, each of her tubes came out, and finally, liberated from the ventilator, she could speak. I tried to laugh about our extensive neurological evaluation for movement disorders that proved to be her simple request for ice. I complimented her ingenuity and ability in communicating with the nurse by using sign language. I chided her for not telling me that she was a communicator with the deaf.

She looked at me as if I were the one exiting a month-long delirium. "I don't know any sign language," she said. "Never have."

As she spoke, her hand started to move in the manner that had so frustrated my diagnostic abilities. The right hand curled with the fingers gently on the palm and the thumb extended. With the mobility of an arm now released from a wrist restraint, she finished the motion and vigorously scratched her nose with her thumb.

A Little Night Poetry

Walter Schmidt, LPN

For the past five years I have been content to work in a nursing home, passing out medications from midnight until dawn. Actually, I had developed a rather pleasant routine that had become as comfortable as a pair of old shoes. I knew, for example, that at 2 o'clock in the morning I would enter room 212 and say, "Wake up, my little pumpkin. It's time for your pill. Down she goes. Atta girl." Then I would continue from room to room, passing out more elixirs, potions, and capsules until I finished my round.

Occasionally, however, I would encounter someone like Emma. She was not the kind who would allow herself to become a part of anyone's routine. This 79-year-old woman insisted that her individuality and personhood be acknowledged at all times. For this reason, many considered Emma to be a difficult patient, and, for this reason, perhaps she was.

On one memorable occasion Emma interrupted my pill-pushing routine with this question: "Do you ever read poetry?" When I replied that I did, she said, "Then I would like to share some of my poems with you," and she handed me a red folder. I opened it and read the dedication to her husband, who had died some years before. The verses that followed dealt with many of the events and concerns of her life, ranging from small philosophical observations she considered while working in her kitchen to the wrenching pain she felt when she lost one of her children forever. It was this sharing, I now realize, that shook the very foundations of my pill-pushing career.

I thought about Emma and her poetry for some time before I considered reading poetry to my patients as I made my rounds. I had not read a poem aloud in years and I wondered what kind of fool my colleagues would think me if I read a poem as I passed a pill. How would my patients respond?

Several weeks passed before I went to the library and checked out a book of poems. I discovered that there were as many wonderful poems to read as there were insomniacs like Emma, awake in the night waiting for a pain pill, or for the sun to rise, or for their God to come take them home.

One evening I slipped a small volume of poems into my pocket along with scissors, tape, and the other tools of my trade. It was 1:30 in the morning when I entered Bill's room and found him wide awake waiting for me. Bill was an old-time Oregonian logger whose arthritis resided around every bone in his body. He was a man's man, I thought, and after giving him his aspirin tablets, I began reading Kipling's "On the Road to Mandalay." When I got to the part about "Ship me somewhere East of Suez, Where the best is like the worst," I glanced up and saw tears in his eyes. Needless to say, I finished reading with a passion that I had not antici-pated. Bill then told me that he used to read poetry when he was a boy. "Robert Service, mostly," he recalled. I said good night to this logger, who suddenly became a sensitive man of substance rather than a receptacle for my pills.

Down the hall was my "little pumpkin" in room 212. Her chart stated that she had once been a schoolteacher but that now she was a victim of Alzheimer's disease. I read to her: "I wandered lonely as a cloud that floats on high o're vales and hills." As I read, she smiled, and when I finished, she said, "Slitherly." I replied, "Good night, Grace." No longer would she be my "little pumpkin."

Perhaps the most moving experience is reading poems to the comatose and dying. "Sleep and rest, Sleep and rest, Father will come to thee soon. Sleep my little one, sleep my pretty one, sleep." They listen. They hear. They know that something very personal is taking place, and so do I. The words seem to cross over the barriers that separate us. It is as if we both reached out into the dark and turned on a light.

Of course, not all of my reading experiences have been so tender or so profound. There was Bonnie, God bless her, who screamed at the top of her voice, as I began reading, "The woods are lovely dark and deep," "Get out of here, you silly son of a bitch, can't you see the house is on fire?" Nor will I soon forget the new patient suffering from acute alcoholism who interrupted "I remember, I remember, the house where I was born" with

"Well goody for you! I can't remember a damn thing!" I know Chester now and realize that he remembers perhaps too much of that which he now tries so hard to forget.

I have found that poems that do their magic best are those that are short and without pretension. Their meaning is clear, direct, and authentic. "I must go down to the seas again, to the lonely seas and the sky." The words ebb and flow with the tide. Some of the most withdrawn people listen to the music of the words even when the words themselves have lost their meaning. It may be that it is the rhythm and pulse of life itself they feel when they hear "For the moon never beams without bringing me dreams of the beautiful Anabel Lee; and the stars never rise but I feel the bright eyes of the beautiful Anabel Lee."

To those who plan to visit a loved one in a nursing home, please give some thought to slipping a book of poems into your pocket. One never knows when the time will be right to read a poem; and if it is, you are sure to have an experience worth remembering.

Taps

Laurie L. Brown, MD

Her first baby died shortly after birth. Her second was stillborn. She desperately wanted a child. Now the time of birth of her third child was near, and she was scheduled for a cesarean section. I was the anesthesiologist.

It was not long after World War II—only a few short years—just enough time for our country to have been involved in another three-year war, commonly known as the Korean conflict. I guess "conflict" doesn't sound as bad as "war," but the thousands who died during that conflict are just as dead as any of those killed in the world's "greatest" wars. Any war is hell on earth! I had finished college and was now in medicine, so I escaped return to active service and another trip to foreign lands.

After the conflict was over, our city remained one of military might. Its uniformed men and women, and its planes and ships and submarines, were ready again to be dispatched at a moment's notice to any place on Earth. A large mine-craft base with its ships and guns and mines and depth charges and other weapons of war was located on the river just across the street from our hospital—a teaching hospital for our state's medical college. It was somehow comforting to look out the operating room windows and see this protection of our freedom so nearby.

Bristling ships of war at a mine-craft base, an anxious patient about to undergo cesarean section: what possible connection could there be?

Erythroblastosis fetalis, then a fairly newly recognized entity, runs the gamut from mild hemolytic anemia of the newborn to permanent brain damage, and often death in utero or shortly after birth. An Rh hemolytic disease, it affects babies born of the union of Rh-negative mothers and Rh-positive fathers. At that time, there was no method of detection or prevention of this dreaded condition. Treatment was symptomatic and consisted of blood transfusions to treat anemia after birth, and often exchange transfusions were used in an attempt to replace damaged red blood cells and with the hope of preventing further hemolysis.

How different it is today: prophylactic administration of Rh immunoglobulin, amniocentesis for early detection of disease severity, early delivery if indicated, and/or intrauterine fetal transfusion with Rh-negative blood.

This brave but apprehensive mother-to-be, hoping against hope that her dream of having a normal baby would now come true, was brought to the operating suite and prepared for spinal anesthesia. General anesthesia wasn't used in such cases for fear that further hemolysis might occur. It was night, and from the seventh floor one could see the dim lights of the nearby ships, which rested ghostlike at anchor.

The spinal anesthetic was given, preparation completed, and the abdominal incision made, quickly followed by opening of the womb. Then came the gush of amniotic fluid—a sickening, thickened, dirty yellow liquid—the sight of which often weakens the knees of the most stoic individual. It was obvious the baby had no chance of life—pallor, hydrops, no cry, no respiration, only a few, short agonal gasps. I went through the motions, but there was no possibility of resuscitation. The mother knew too, but, after a painful hesitation, asked anyway. As I nodded my head and held her hand, hoping to be of some slight comfort, the beautiful but oh! so mournful strains of *Taps*, played by the bugler down the river, sounded achingly clear throughout the quiet night. "My God!" was heard faintly from the surgeon. "Oh no, oh no, oh no!" sobbed the mother. As I whispered "I'm sorry," I kissed her gently on the forehead, and quickly eased her into sleep, postponing for her all too briefly one of the real tragedies of life—which so many of our patients suffer, and which we so often share during the practice of medicine.

The View From Here

I believe there is a place for patients' stories in a medical journal, even if some readers react with surprise that *JAMA* allows nonphysicians' writings on its pages. But many readers have told me that these articles are some of the most helpful and enlightening we publish, giving them a chance to experience what it's like on the other side, or even an opportunity to see how a colleague handled a particularly difficult situation. In "He Lifted His Eyes," for example, a mother is grateful—and slightly stunned—when her daughter's exhausted physician notices the child's fear of an impending procedure and shows remarkable insight, feeling, compassion, and commiseration. In "Windows," a man with advanced throat cancer decides to discontinue therapy, concluding that treatment will only interfere with such basic but now-cherished activities as enjoying sunny windows. Occasionally, physicians and medical students try to put themselves in their patients' shoes. In "The Venetian Blinds," a medical student imagines the thoughts of a man who is told he will need a respirator permanently. The patient strikes out and tries to end his existence by pulling out his lifesaving breathing line; but his plan is foiled by his caregivers who return him to life support. These essays reiterate that only when we've walked in another's shoes can we truly "see things through his eyes."

R.K.Y.

Pace, Pace

Naomi G. Smith

She hadn't the entourage at her deathbed that my father had had. Only me, and I wasn't there at the end. Finally left, stopping on the way home to buy a sandwich, barely sitting down in front of the TV to eat it before the phone rang.

"I'm sorry, your mother is dead," the nurse said. Pause. "I think she waited until you'd left."

I felt a vast, encompassing wave of relief. It was tinged with regret that I hadn't stayed just a little longer, but mostly there was relief.

The whole thing had gone on for so long and I was so tired. Sometimes I felt that maybe I was as tired of it as she, tired of watching her battered by the strokes that nibbled at her faculties, destroying a muscle here, a nerve center there, blurring her speech, the cruel little stroke that sliced her sight, leaving each eye half-seeing, half-blind. She had become enclosed in her infirmities.

Sitting at her bedside those long months, I'd flinched at the rage that howled from those damaged eyes, berating the world for its unfairness, berating me for not being able to help her. I became adept at translation, at seeing what she could not say, seeing love, and flashes of humor, a self-pity that left me impatient and annoyed, and then, sometimes, I saw a rueful resignation that caught me unaware and tore my heart more than her rage, her humor, more even than her love.

My mother and father had grown enfeebled at different rates, like leaves wafting past each other in a gentle downward spiral in which one would suddenly hit a gust that would carry it past the other. It was my father whose incapacities first necessitated entering a nursing home, Mother still able to wash her best china and set out silver for the ladies who came to afternoon coffee. When Mother finally faltered, however, the change was breathtaking, and she came to that same nursing home needing more care than my father.

But during the next months, though separated by two floors and antiseptic halls, they saw each other nearly every day. Either I or my sisters would take one to visit the other, push Dad's wheelchair up to Mother's room or take Mother down to Dad. Between the deafness of one, the other's aphasia, and their diminished capacity for speech, they could not understand each other. But they held hands. When Mother wept, as sometimes she did, my father would reach out and pat her shoulder. His own initial anger, his frustrated rage at finding himself helpless, beholden for every need, had long since quieted to an acceptance that enabled him to find joy in the small things that now made up his life.

Throughout the long day when my father died, they had been together. Mother, her wheelchair by his bed, held his hand as I read to them. Read psalms and parables and revelations of a life to come, those passages my father, a minister, had often read to others. Then later, when it seemed that there would indeed be an ending to his endless lassitude, there had been time for others to join us. Time even for the moment when, alerted by his physician grandson that death was near, we all held hands and said the Lord's Prayer. His pulse stopped, our son said, as we uttered the "Amen." It was an easing into death that seemed, in retrospect, sweet as honey.

Mother survived, for a while. She came to his funeral service, her wheelchair at the front of the church beside the first pew. There, propped against cushions and listing to one side, she'd wailed a soaring, indistinct counterpart to the hymns, her inarticulateness unchained for this brief period, no longer an old woman in a bed with bars on the sides, but again part of a world from which she had been wrested by age and infirmity.

After the service she clutched the hands that reached out to clasp hers, nodding and smiling as though this were one of the church socials she'd so often attended. It was as though she celebrated the rite of passage whose secret initiations she now knew. And then she held court at the family gathering that followed, responding with gracious garbled speech to the grandchild, the son, the daughter who came to kneel beside her chair.

But that was the end. Within days she had another "episode," as they called the seizures, and after that there was only lethargy, disinterest, and a gentle drift away from us. Not even the mention of her grandchildren, those precious extensions of her life, could rouse her from her torpor.

———————

"Your mother's not doing well."

It wasn't the first time I'd been called to her side to watch and wait. And this was much like other times, so when I phoned the family it was only to say that Mother was having a bad day.

I sat beside her bed, read her some of those same psalms I'd read four months earlier in my father's room, held her hand as she had held his. Sat and listened to her heavy, labored breathing as she sucked in air that rattled obscenely in her throat and then exited with little whooshing noises. Sat and wondered how long the frail body could keep up this battle for air. Asked the nurse if something could be done and when, calm and efficient, she aspirated Mother and the breathing immediately eased, took my place beside the bed again. And after a while, looking out over the angled rooftops of the nursing home, I sang.

Hymns, those songs she'd sung throughout her long life, the years of her girlhood, the 60 years of her marriage, and as I sang, the air she sucked in and breathed out changed pitch, rising and falling with the notes. At first I wasn't sure, but when I stopped, so did she. Singing softly, I began again, touched with wonder, accompanied by her sighing song.

When the nurse came in the room I stopped, self-conscious, but Mother, in the swing of things now, breathed an accompaniment to the music of her roommate's TV. "Listen to that," said the nurse. "She's trying to sing Happy Birthday, right?"

"Right," I said.

And when we were alone again, we sang some more.

"Let go," I whispered at last. "It's all right, you can let go."

But she didn't. So I went home and stopped to pick up my sandwich on the way, not knowing that somewhere between Dempster Street and Burnham Court my mother's song had stilled.

The Great Wait

Janice F. Lalikos, MD

12:30 PM

"The surgeon said they'd be done between 4 and 5."

"But the anesthesiologist said it might be after 6."

"I think he meant it might be 6 before we can see him."

"Do you want a Coke or something? . . . I need a cold drink. . . . Can I get you anything while I'm up?"

I have started counting the pin-holed ceiling tiles. They have stale coffee-colored stains in the corners from age. Like a miniature Venetian hedge garden, the green vinyl chairs are arranged in discrete geometric patterns with round wooden tables speckled throughout, stacked with outdated news of "Liz's Marriage," "Baseball's Winter Training," and "Twelve Low-Fat Quickbreads." Next to me, a woman with noticeably applied makeup begins talking without introduction—very animated— not like she's initiating a discussion, but as if she is continuing aloud her previously silent train of thought.

"You know," she starts. I place my magazine on my lap. "The lady volunteer at that desk with the orange smock on. She says she has the same gynecologist as my daughter has. Well, she thinks he's wonderful. I certainly hope so. He said it would only take two hours or so, unless they found something bad. But he said it didn't look bad on the sonny-gram, like a cyst, a four-by-five cyst. Four-by-five seems big to me. But he made it sound easy. I hope he's right. Doesn't that sound big? What do I know?" She shifts uncomfortably in her chair and continues talking, just to talk.

I look across my coffee table and see a gray-haired man in a well-tailored wool coat peering over his morning edition of the *Globe*, straining to hear her conversation. He seems to be seeking some solace for his own private anxiety.

A young child, diagonally across in another sitting unit, is restless and impatient. Despite his parents' repeated warnings to behave, the boy shrieks and stomps on the floor; a short outburst that, for a moment, halts all other activity in the room. But, after a pause, people resume reading, some leaning, in synchrony, toward their respective coffee tables to change magazines. One or two others drift to the condiment area and linger, mixing the perfect cup of tepid instant coffee with prepackaged powdered milk substitute. And we all wait.

My mother has come back with her Coke but doesn't drink it. Three months ago, she lost her sister to cancer. Then, my father suffered a heart attack, and now requires coronary artery bypass grafting. She has been reassured by the experts that his prognosis is excellent and that his surgical course should be smooth. But there are no guarantees. Watching her nervously wait, I wonder if she's strong enough to hear any more bad news.

2 PM

"Janice, you never knew your grandfather, did you? He was a wonderful man. He looked just like your father, 'cept with more curly hair on top and a little mustache. A proud, quiet, Greek man." My aunt is talking with exaggerated hand gestures and emphatic nods, gathering the attention of those around us. They all begin nodding too, as if they knew my grandfather. "You know he lost his arm in the leather factory," she continues. The audience nods. They knew. "But Janice, that never stopped him. Brave, full of life— just like your dad is—right through the Depression."

My mother is smiling weakly, half-listening, staring at the flower prints hanging on the laminated paneling. She has noticed that one picture is not straight and wants desperately to correct it. Her Coke is stale. She throws it away.

A physician stops at the volunteer's desk and briefly questions the attendant. She points out the wool-coated gentleman in our section. The surgeon strides quickly to his side and begins telling him in perfunctory terms that his wife's hernia operation "went off without a hitch." The community leans in to hear the outcome and breathes a unified sigh as they see the relief on the man's face. When the surgeon leaves, the man folds his paper in half under his arm and saunters out of the area, restraining himself from skipping. Everyone envies him. A few whispers of "Thank God" are heard as he leaves. Then we all resume talking, reading, pacing, or dozing.

3:30 PM

Four weather-beaten workmen scuffle into the stuffy sanctuary. Their mountain boots are crusted with mud and each man has a beard that probably gets trimmed only on special occasions. There is one small woman among them, with puffy, red-rimmed eyes. Her husband has been flown in with extensive damage from a wood chipper. The group instinctively marks out a territory on the left side of the room with their down-stuffed parkas and Igloo coolers. The volunteer approaches them and states, "His operation may take as long as 15 hours. Would you like me to arrange some lodging for you?" They shake their heads no, and the oldest, in a red flannel shirt, mumbles that they will stay here. Soon they are settled, except for one man who is sent out as a scout to find the cafeteria.

My neighbor has yet to hear about her daughter. At some point she discovers that I am interested in plastic surgery. She barrages me with legal questions about silicone breast prostheses. She argues her beliefs, quoting *People* magazine and *The Ladies Home Journal*. I defend the surgeon's perspective, outlining current scientific evidence. However, I soon realize that she (and I) are tiring of the discourse and it winds down. Our hearts are just not in it.

After a few minutes, she blurts out, "How does it feel to get a taste of your own medicine?" With a regal wave of her arm, she motions me to gaze about the anguished, uncomfortable room. There is a hint of vindictiveness in her voice. I do not answer, but I know what she is feeling. Hours of uncertainty. Hours of helplessness. Hours of silence. There is a heavy, suffocating fatigue in this confined area, a tangible awareness of time, and its ability to torment.

5 PM

Now my mother's gaze is fixed on the telephone atop the volunteer's desk. She is not the only one. When the phone rings, the room freezes. If a physician comes to the suite, half a dozen people stand at attention, ready for the verdict. We all know each other now, maybe not by name, but we are tethered together on the same tension wire. A gastrectomy, a digital replant, a brain tumor, a bypass. The titles are like powerful scenes in a daytime drama. And we, as uninvited guests, must patiently perch at the stage door, praying for a happy ending.

Finally, at 5:30 PM, my mother is called into a small adjacent consultation room. The volunteer closes the door behind them. A few deafening seconds pass and then my mother reappears—elated. "He's out of surgery," she pronounces. "He is in the cardiac intensive care unit. He has had two bypasses and he's OK." She is beaming; the great "wait" has been lifted. The congregation is happy for her. With congratulations completed, we move quickly now; my mother, my aunt, and myself. We call several selected family members and then hurry out of the surgical waiting area, wishing well to the ones remaining. It has been seven hours too long.

The next morning, when we are together again, this time in the intensive care visiting area, I ask my mother what impressed her the most about yesterday.

She begins. "It seemed like one of the longest days of my life." She pauses, then adds, "Interestingly enough, I remember the cleaning lady. She had a sweatshirt with a curse word printed on it. She didn't seem to care that it offended all those families." After pondering my question further, my mother says, "Also, I wondered why my doctor called me on the phone instead of coming down to talk to me like some of the other doctors. I guess he was just too busy." She concludes, "I hope that that lady's daughter, the lady in the dark dress who was sitting next to you, I hope her daughter is well."

I hope so too.

Thirty Years Later

Norma C. Wark

Wait there on the examining table, please, Mrs Wark. The doctor will be with you in a few minutes." With these familiar words, the nurse left us alone—my pounding heart, my apprehensive thoughts, and my dissembling ego. My pounding heart and my apprehensive thoughts always force my ego to dissemble whenever I am waiting for the doctor.

Perched there, disrobed from the waist up, as ordered, I heard my facetious thoughts interject, "Do you think Rodin's afflatus for his famous *Thinker* occurred in the doctor's examining room while he mused about whether a pounding heart precipitates apprehensive thoughts or apprehensive thoughts precipitate a pounding heart? Something like the chicken and the egg quandary," they concluded.

The resolution of this cause-and-effect problem would have to wait. The booming of my heart was beginning to resound around the Naval Hospital examining room, disturbing its silence.

"I apologize for this booming," my heart sighed, "but it seems that we have been waiting for a long time, and I am getting a little nervous. Will we be waiting much longer?"

A few reassuring words for all of us might help, I hoped. "Pay attention, please. Everything is going to be fine. It is just a checkup. We have been having one every year for the last 30, and each time since that memorable year of '62 we have been given another lease on life."

"Uh huh!" entered my insistent apprehensive thoughts. "But what if in their checkup this time they find something that will cancel the lease? And what about all those new questions from this new doctor? New doctors and new questions sometimes bring new problems. Furthermore, your pounding heart is exacerbating my worrying."

"I believe you are in error," throbbed my heart. "It is your apprehensive thinking that is exacerbating my excitable pulsating."

"Please listen!" I scolded. "Neither one of you is paying attention. I repeat, everything is going to be fine!"

"I must find some way to keep them quiet before I have a stroke," I counseled myself.

"Time for a little dissembling," my aware thoughts interposed. I began, "This is not my heart, these are not my thoughts, these are not my mastectomies, these are not my scars, this is not my skin graft . . ."

"Hello!" The new young doctor's greeting brought us all to attention. "Well," he began, as he perused my folder with its extensive medical history, "140 pounds—good weight. I see your pressure is a little high. Are you taking your pills?" I nodded yes. He continued, "Feeling well?"

"Oh yes," I answered promptly with enthusiasm so he would know that there was nothing wrong with me. "I'm feeling fine."

"That's good." He smiled as he placed my bulky folder on the table. "Do you work or are you retired?" he asked, sort of conversationally it seemed to me.

"Both," I answered sort of conversationally. "I'm retired from the New England Telephone Company, but now I teach the children of the second grade."

"Hmmm," he murmured, as he continued his examination, "has your skin graft ever broken down?" That calm attitude I had convinced myself was mine was shattered, but I answered, insouciantly, I hoped, "No."

"What do you mean, 'no'? You don't even know what he is talking about!" my shocked thoughts exclaimed. Then they added tersely, "If he asks any more questions like that, *we* are going to break down!"

"Sh, sh," I warned them, "the graft has remained the same all these years so it must not have broken down . . ."

"Radical mastectomy on the left breast and simple of the right," the doctor continued. "Cancer?"

"He certainly didn't read the important part," I heard muttered. But I staccatoed as usual, "Yes, of my left but prophylactic of the right."

Then, as always, after giving those sensitive data, I was taking a deep breath . . . "We don't *do* prophylactics now," the doctor informed me casually, and looking at me as though *I* had made the decision (without giving it too much thought), he inquired, "Was the radical necessary?"

The suspension of my vital signs precluded my answering, so he did. "You know, research has shown that many of these operations were and are unnecessary." (I had heard about it but never suspected it might apply to my operation.) "But," he smiled (as a palliative afterthought, I am sure), "you are still here, so we could say it was successful, if not necessary."

"We can live with that," spoke up my facetious thoughts. "We never did like the one about the operation that was a success but the patient died. But what are you going to do about knowing that this research is 30 years too late?"

"We will talk about it later," I cautioned them sternly. But I smiled my thank-you happily to the very young doctor when again I heard those blessed words, "Everything looks fine, no evidence of any recurrence. See you next year, unless you have any problems before then."

Problems! Finding the answer to his question "Was the operation necessary?" was an immediate problem. My mind, like earth in space, was going around in circles. I left the hospital and walked on automatic to the parking area.

When I reached and started my car, I realized that I was still operating on automatic, so I turned the motor off and left the shift in the park position. "Better I park here until my equilibrium is restored than be brought back to the hospital, ironically, as an accident statistic," I advised myself wisely.

"And speaking of statistics," my attentive thoughts reminded me, "remember, you are one."

"Yes, I am one," I repeated. "A cured-of-breast-cancer statistic. Thank you for bringing it to my attention. It seems I do need to be reminded occasionally." I sighed gratefully. To express my gratitude, should I give life to this sterile statistic? Should I resurrect and relive my lonely fears, and doubts, my physical and psychological pain? Should I write about these poignant memories, offering them as hope for someone?

Since these questions were asked of no one in particular, my heart answered, "Maybe if your story leads someone to an answer to what might be an inexpressible, painful question, shouldn't you try? And maybe in the reliving of those old, agonizing questions, their revealing answers, and your final victory, you will find the answer to today's poignant question, "Was the operation necessary?"

"Thank you, dear heart, we know she'll write it now," answered my thoughts so excitedly that the pursuance of an alternative was precluded.

I turned the key in the ignition, started the car, and drove home. Having arrived there safely, I was searching, trying to find in my memory bank a beginning to my story when my now cooperating thoughts suggested, "Why don't you start with the first question you asked the doctor upon wakening after the operation?"

My heart whispered, "It is going to be difficult, but the remembrance of the love, beauty, and compassion of those who answered your questions then will give you the courage you need to start, and the rest of the story will just unfold."

So I resurrected my first question, and my caring doctor's tender but shocking answer. "Why do I hurt so much on my left side?" I had asked, conscious only of the pain there, and of the compassion reflected in his eyes when he had to answer, "I am so sorry we had to remove your breast—it was cancer. We are sure we got all of it."

It took only the moment needed—before I returned to the welcome womb of darkness—to ask the question, "May I see my mother? Please!"

Upon awakening again, I asked my mother, who was there beside me in the intensive care unit, Job's universal question, "Why? Why me, Mama?" And from her grief-stricken heart she answered, "I don't know, Norma, I wish I did. I would change places with you if only I could." The pain in her heart was reflected in her tear-filled eyes, as the pain in her body was reflected in the misshapen arthritic hand with which she held mine. With her hand enclosing mine as if she were taking my pain to herself, I entered again the darkness of nonsuffering.

The memory of the pain is no longer with me, but the memory of the young corpsman and his answer to my question upon awakening will remain with me for my lifetime. "Please, must you massage or do whatever it is you are doing?" I pleaded. "It hurts so." And with understanding and compassion coming from his young soul, he answered, "Yes, I must. I'm sorry I have to hurt you, but it will be over soon; you are going to be all right; don't cry, don't cry; you are going to be fine. Trust in God, trust Him." May that young humanitarian find someone as caring as himself if ever he has the need.

My loving husband's answer is not just a memory. I live with it every day. By my side day and night for the six weeks that I remained in the hospital, he waited with his answer to the question he knew I had to ask. "Am I all right? Am I all right for you? I am no longer a complete woman." With his love reaching and touching mine, he answered, "You will always be all right for me. There is nothing that can happen that will change my feelings for my woman."

My doctor's excitement and joy in calling out to me while I was in the shower can never be just a memory. Not being able to wait with such wonderful news, he was shouting through the door, "Mrs Wark! Mrs Wark! Can you hear me? Can you hear me? The tests are back! Everything's fine! Everything's fine!" These words, and my doctor who called them out, are part of the "me" who welcomes each day because of them.

Very often, when I am pulling my cart on the golf course while enjoying my long hundred-yard drives and Florida's tropical breezes, I relive the memory of my nurse's answer. "OK," she would say, "time to climb that wall with those fingers."

"Do I have to?" I would ask. "It's not much fun, you know." Then laughingly she would say, "If you want to get out on that golf course and swing away with those clubs, you had better start swinging away now with your arm; come on now, start climbing. It hurts a little but like your golf game, it will get better each day."

And she was right about my arm. It is better. I wish, however, when I am alone in the woods looking for my lost ball, that she was right about my golf game.

My heart was right, as usual. In the kindness of the doctors who worked so skillfully that I might have life, and in the concern of all those whose lives touched mine during my painful intimacy with bitterness, I found my answer. I found it in the inherent dignity of humankind; the dignity that someone's need had unveiled.

I saw it in the caring doctor's compassionate eyes. I touched it in my loving mother's hands. I felt it in my faithful husband's understanding. I enjoyed it in my nurse's authoritative humor. I heard it in the excited doctor's joy when he couldn't wait to say those precious words, "Everything's fine! Everything's fine!" and in the sensitive young corpsman's sadness when he cried his comforting ultimate words, "Don't cry, don't cry, trust Him, trust Him."

Conceived in the dignity of humankind, this language of compassion offered me, and I embraced, the peace of its answer to my tormenting question, "Why? Why me?"

Our being, our humanness, is the embodiment of all the answers to questions whose essence is "Why?"

I rejoice in my being, my humanness.

I cherish these moments that are uniquely mine.

I behold the mosaic of my life within which is my answer for today as it was my answer for all my yesterdays, and shall be for all my tomorrows, and I am grateful.

I live my gratitude.

I am the answer.

"Amen!" sing my heart and my thoughts.

Epilogue

"Hi, dear," Sterling called as he came in the door. "Everything all right at the doctor's office?"

I looked at my husband, whose love for me and mine for him is now 40 years old, but forever young, and answered, insouciantly, "The new young doctor asked a few poignantly provoking questions, but everything is still fine—no problems!"

What Are We Going to Do About Mother?

Evalynn Morgan Quisenberry, BFA

Martha means well. It's just that she has been doing some pretty crazy things lately. I've been wanting to tell the doctor every time we go. But, as usual, Martha does all the talking for both of us. I don't talk much at all anymore, but I keep thinking about what I want to say.

Martha called in the burglar alarm people. She told them she wanted to install a system for keeping people in the house, not for keeping people out. They were as puzzled as I was.

Next time I really will speak up; I'll tell the doctor. This latest thing Martha did really has me bugged. She bought a small green bath mat and put it by the front door. She told me it was a hole and if I stepped on it I'd fall in. I don't think a sane person would say that.

The doctor told me there was something wrong with my depth perception way back when I was told I couldn't drive the car anymore. But that little rug is flat as a pancake. I was with Martha when she bought it at the bathroom store. I sure hate shopping, always have. Now she takes me every time whether I want to go or not. I used to stay home and watch TV or look at the newspapers while she was gone.

Then the day came when the table with the yellow flowers fell over. I tried to clean it up but I cut my hand on the broken glass. There was red all over the place. When Martha came home she found me at the sink trying to stop the bleeding with hot water. She turned off the faucet and put my hand in a bowl of ice. I had to carry it on my lap while the taxi took us to the doctor to get sewed up. She cried a little and told the doctor she didn't think I could turn on the faucet. (I have trouble with things like that. Now I can't do buttons or doorknobs or light switches or turn on the stove.)

Martha talks to the doctor about me as if I wasn't there or as if I can't hear. It's embarrassing, but they won't wait for me to talk.

When we got home I showed Martha how I saved her flowers. I put them in the fish tank. Then Martha told me that wasn't the kind of flowers that needed water, when there is dirt on the roots. She was very calm; sometimes she yells her head off. Martha is not a swearing woman but I sure don't like it when she shouts at me.

I really made her mad one day this week. She was all excited about company coming and she was busy cooking in the kitchen. She set the big, long dining room table with white linen and sterling flatware and our wedding crystal. Flowers from the florist were in the middle, with six candles.

She let me get dressed by myself for once. I can do it, I'm just slow; she puts everything out for me so I don't have to search for stuff. I got my shoes and socks on by myself. She does too much for me anyway. She even runs my zipper up and down for me. I was proving to myself that I could do it alone but as soon as the zipper was down I got the strong urge to urinate. I didn't know what to do. I wasn't in the bathroom, but there was the open drawer.

Boy, you could sure hear some fancy screaming and yelling that time, I tell you.

"Charles, what have you done?" she said and kept on talking loud. She sure was mad when she saw the water running out of the drawer onto the carpet. She always calls me Charles. Other people call me Charlie or Chuck.

While she was cleaning up and making all that noise, I decided to go out. The round rug was still there but I went around the edges just in case. I couldn't remember where I had to go but I knew it would come to me if I kept walking.

I used to walk a lot for exercise. Nowadays I'm not as sure-footed as I used to be. I never get turned around or lost and I always look for street signs and traffic signs, but I don't see them like I used to. The traffic seems heavier than usual; there is a lot of honking, shouting, and screeching brakes, especially at intersections. People are more rude than they used to be. One man showed me his dirty finger.

I must have walked a long way before I came to the park where I could sit down. I was thirsty. I couldn't get the drinking fountain handle to work. I started to get cold. I wished I had my sweater. It was warm enough while

I was walking but I got chilly just sitting there. I think it is November. There are turkey decorations in the store windows.

One of the fellows in the park asked if I didn't want something to eat. I hate it when somebody comes up alongside me like that. I think I'm being attacked. When he came in front of me where I could see him it was OK. It's like looking down a tunnel sometimes.

I was sure hungry, all right. I guess I walked a couple hours or more; I was ready to drop. They put me in some kind of van with some others and let us all out at a big hall where there were long paper-covered tables and folding chairs. There was a lady wearing an old-fashioned bonnet playing a piano on a stage. A man in a uniform was playing a guitar and singing into a microphone. I think the song was the old hymn "Bringing in the Sheaves."

I remembered how pretty Martha had set our table at home and I thought I should be there.

They gave me a big plate of stuff and I was hungry but I couldn't eat. Looking at all that food overwhelmed me. Martha just gives me one thing at a time.

Then the other guys started asking me for the food off my plate that I wasn't eating, but I didn't care as long as I had some soda pop.

I looked down at the end of the hall and saw some policemen. Then I recognized my daughter-in-law Lottie standing with them.

"Hi, Charlie, I've come to take you home." She walked over to put some coins in the phone and left me with the two young officers. They talked about me as if I wasn't there. I hate that. They were speaking about me in the past tense as if I were already dead.

Lottie and I got in the back of the squad car and the boys played the siren all the way home. I didn't say anything but I liked it.

Martha looked just awful. Her hair needed combing and her face was puffy and red as if she had been crying. Usually she puts on a little lipstick when we have company. She didn't get up out of her chair. She looked old and pale. She was holding baby Linda, who was asleep. All our kids were there and the grandkids were on the floor in front of the TV.

Wilbur took me to the bathroom and then got me ready for bed. I like a tub bath but Martha can't lift me, so we shower. She gets right in with me. She says she can't soap me up past the shower curtain without getting all wet herself so she might as well get in.

I sure did sleep that night, you bet. The next morning Martha was back to her old tricks again. She had put a strip of masking tape across the floor in front of the door. She thinks it is some kind of barrier.

Touch Me

Meg Verrees

I am alone. I am alone and I am lonely. I am very sick, though not too old, and I believe that I am here in the hospital for the last time. I am weak. I am tired. I am alone. I am alone not because I lived carelessly or was thoughtless. I was never stingy or sour or mean. I never cheated anyone or profited from a neighbor's misfortune. I was never knowingly cruel, never spiteful. I never intentionally deceived anyone, man or woman. All my life I never took advantage of innocence. I am alone. I am alone now as I have always been alone. But this is the first time I have been lonely.

As a poet I lived invariably surrounded by penciled proof of my thoughts, my ideas. I passed the time enveloped by my own creation of reality. I strove to unearth some hint of charm in each situation. But I can find no beauty in dying alone. Beauty has abandoned me, as has laughter. Only the reality of this room is left. And truth unaccompanied by grace or happiness is a chilly friend.

The walls girding this room rise stark and narrow. Alternating rows of beige and white threads form the skirt flanking the far, recessed window. The bed sheets are ivory and stiff. The closed door to this place is carved from a square of blanched wood. A spare, frosted bulb hangs above me. To the wall sticks a drawing of a seashell—pale pink lines on bleached paper. Behind a pane of glass one hump of grainy cloud strains the elegant azure streaks of the sky.

My skin is pale. The nurses who hastily enter and exit this place cloak in pale smocks. Their hands remain the waxen white of the rubber gloves they wear when they touch me. Each time they strip off the slippery coverings, before they wash their hands under the faucet in the corner, I see the sheath of white powder that tightly clings to rough skin. The dusty film rims the insides of the gloves. The women stoop over the sink and knead their palms with their fingertips until a balloon of plump lather encases their fists. They repeat this soaping three or four times. Then they rinse for a long while. I hear the water slurp down the drain. For a few moments each morning, a group of doctors stands at the foot of my bed. These do not touch me at all. They mumble among themselves and mispronounce my name.

I am alone. I am alone and I am lonely. I am too high here on the eighth floor to see any life, to see children jumping off schoolbuses, to see mothers pushing baby carriages or eye business folk rushing from stoplight to stoplight on their way to work or to important appointments. I cannot witness bicyclists wedge fair riding space between tough strings of traffic and snapped ribbons of curb. I cannot watch the packed 8-o'clock buses rush by or see the off-hour shuttles boasting only five passengers: two seated in the rear, a pair fogging windows in the middle, and a chatty soul entrenched behind the driver. I cannot spy any trees. I lie high above even the highest boughs. The birds stay away from my corner pane. There must be no ledge outside the glass for them to rest. Missing is a perch for them to linger.

The air between these walls hangs empty, devoid of any scent, different from sky filled with the redolence of freshly cut grass or baking bread. Or the smell of raindrops falling on warm stalks of wheat. No one leans close enough to share some fragrance of humanity—perfume or lotion or sweat.

Last night a ball of crushed paper towel fell into the path of the door, leaving the wooden flange propped slightly away from its frame, exposing a slice of hallway life for me to view—strips of movement rippling past like the shaded streamers of a tall barber pole or scored designs of a whirling totem. A man with a curly beard and silver tooth strode along, followed by a woman with gooey red lipstick towing a youth clad in a pair of stretchy, black-and-white checkered pants. A kitchen aide raced past shoving a cart of soiled trays. A raunchy laugh from afar interrupted the incessant decency of a nearby whispered bedside conversation.

A housekeeper entered the room to polish the floor. First she pushed her broom across the tiles in broad, heavy strokes. Next she leaned against the wooden stick and stared out the window. Lucky woman—to stand by the ledge and peer over the sill and absorb life from what must be a teeming courtyard far below. But her eyes remained dour, ignoring the animation I imagined must meet her gaze. She rested her head against the glass, leaving a smudge on the pane. She rubbed the thickened ends of her fingertips over her face. Then she turned away from the window and again set to work, leaning into each swipe of the broom, scooping the wad of paper towel wedged in the path of the door.

At the end of the job she sighed and at the threshold began to peel away the garb she had donned as she entered my place. She reached with her bare fist for the metal door handle. In a few seconds she would vanish, taking with her the stripe of light, the lady marked with bright lipstick, and the sailor with jaw outlined by wide beard, disappear with the kitchen clerk hoisting trays and the reluctant lad outfitted in snappy pants. The maid turned the knob and with the swoosh of door opening a few twerpy strings of hall wind stirred the imprisoned core of room air.

I forced myself upright in bed and cleared my throat. She loosened her grip on the door and turned toward me, startled. Surprise brightened her eyes. Charmed, naive eyes. "Did you know . . . did you know I tell fortunes?" I whispered—a flip, bald-faced lie. Her shoulders turned farther inward, deeper into the room, away from the hall. Life played in those eyes. "I tell fortunes," I remarked without shame. My rusty voice scratched the emptiness, squelched the quick, flexing spirit of guilt. I stretched one hand across my chest to trace the swooping lines of the resting palm with one finger.

The woman paused a fair moment but then took steps toward my space on the bed. She found a platter-smooth square of mattress, just next to me, and held out one unshielded hand. I grasped her unfurling fingers and touched the frayed, blistered skin and torn callouses. I tried not to seem desperate, too insatiably wanting. I examined the creases and told the woman that all in her life would be well. I told her that with effort everything through the years would work out for the best. I thought of the words my mother had offered me when I was little—true or false—the whispered reassurances I wished she could step into the room and repeat that minute. I recycled a few gritty tales my father had shared when I lost at school games or at play fell wounded. I wrenched from dim memory the maxims teachers had extended to calm me when I felt small and defeated. And these seemed to please her. The smoky pall veiling her face effervesced. Her countenance brightened. She explained her problems and I listened. My eyelids sagged but one last ounce of will trussed them open, not daring to squander the moment. We talked. I kept tight hold of her hand. Then I let her go. Exhausted, I lay back against the blankets. Evening came, and I fell asleep in the room.

I am alone. I am alone and I am lonely. I hold one of my hands in the other, to feel some warmth. But my hands are cold. I grasp my left wrist with my right hand. I rub the fingers of my left hand over my right arm. I must touch myself to feel any warmth because no one else will touch me without the gloves. Everyone is afraid of me.

I am alone and I am dying and everything is pale around me. I am cold. I am weak. I have spent my life writing my thoughts, my visions, my ideas. But I am now too spent to place, or even to imagine, these last thoughts on paper. Most of my work is known only to me, and so will these last thoughts be mine alone.

I am alone. I am alone and I am lonely. I have one desire. I have one hope. I hope that someone, anyone, will remove one glove and hold my hand before I die. I hope that someone will come in and sit by my side and take off one glove and touch my hand. I hope that someone will take off one glove—just for a moment—and touch me.

Respect for the Dead

Dian G. Smith

K'vod ha-met: in Hebrew, respect for the dead. For Jews, this ancient principle ensures dignified treatment of the body. Even in liberal Judaism, only certain conditions can override it: when civil law requires an autopsy, for example, to determine the cause of death; or when there is an opportunity to save a life.

When my mother died, there was no question about the cause. Her death certificate may read "heart failure" or "pneumonia" (I never looked), but she died of multiple sclerosis. She had been wasted by a devastating disease. Literally wasted.

The moment I hung down the telephone from the caller telling me that she was dead, I opened my top desk drawer. I took out the folded clipping I had guarded there for over two years, hidden at the back. I dialed the number of a doctor at a medical school in California. "Do you still need brain tissue from MS patients?" That was all. The rest would be handled discreetly, antiseptically, hospital-to-hospital.

But still I had to ask my brother. I had to admit to him that I had planned that telephone call for two years, that for me the woman who had been our mother was long dead. He was appalled and angry. How could it matter? he insisted. It was indecent. He consented finally, but only on condition that the procedure not alter her appearance. Why did he want to see her body anyway, and remember her like that?

I knew how I wanted to remember her. In that same desk drawer I kept a photographic slide fit into a tiny pink satin pocket. Although I never saw it projected, I had held it up to the light countless times. As a child, I kept it in a wooden box bound with ribbon, which contained all my most secret and sacred treasures. I took it to sleepaway camp with me as an amulet, to ward off night fears and homesickness, and I brought it to my marriage as a memento.

The slide is over 40 years old now, its cardboard frame browned and bent, but the image is still bright and clear. A young woman, small and slim, with soft dark curls, wearing a red-and-white striped shirt and blue shorts in an athletic pose. She reaches her arm behind her head as if to throw the tennis ball in her hand. She didn't know yet. I can tell by the carefree smile. I remember when she stopped playing tennis, and I remember when she stopped smiling.

Some people count their blessings; my mother counted her losses. They came slowly at first, like little nasty pinches of the flesh from a spiteful demon. One month she lost some feeling in her hand (foreshadowed by the "tingling" she came to dread); the next month the feeling came back, almost. One month she limped; the next she could walk almost as well as before. One month her eyesight blurred; the next month she saw clearly but needed glasses.

The almosts and buts of her body began to mount and weigh her down. The indignities grew also. Her hand twitched whenever she wasn't looking directly at it. She phoned me from Florida to tell me that. "I was at the airport in Portland," she told me the next time. "I had to make a connection, to get from one gate to another. I knew I had to run. But I couldn't do it." She missed her flight. I didn't know what to say so I said nothing.

In a restaurant she asked me to come with her to the ladies' room. She had wet her underpants. She was immobilized with shame. Silently I put the pants in the wastebasket, gave her mine, and we returned to the table—both terrified by her incontinence. Already this was more than I could bear to know so I stopped knowing. Finally, in its relentless course, the disease invaded her mind, leaving only a teasing shadow to lie in bed for ten long years.

There was no silver lining, no moral lesson, no nobility in my mother's illness. She did not rise to face it with either courage or grace. My father couldn't summon the emotional powers necessary to comfort her. He found the best doctors, supported the most promising research, read the latest studies. Then, beaten and broken-hearted, he died. Medical science offered her no miracles and scant hope. I was too self-centered and frightened myself to hear her cries, or my father's. The disease that should have pulled us close as a family instead walled us apart.

That is why I saved the clipping—to salvage something out of respect for her. Now I cherish articles about the first new drug being used to treat MS. I strain for news of people who are taking it. Does it work? I need to know. The drug itself may not have come from the lab in California, but still it is my mother's legacy: that bit of diseased tissue from her brain, which tormented and killed her, is helping to save lives.

K'vod ha-met.

A Thin Green Line

Scott Waters

Today I saw my father's heart.

It was a glowing green line on a monitor in the naval air station hospital intensive care unit. Early this morning his prostate had been removed, along with a battalion of adventurous cells that had dared to become cancerous without his permission.

The tiny line squiggled along, dropped to a narrow notch, then zoomed back up to resume formation. After a dozen repetitions, the line disappeared and began again, marching across the screen from left to right in a stubbornly consistent procession of green phosphors.

On the bed, a thin, gray man slept, pierced by transparent tubes and wrapped in clean, white linen. His thin, gray hair stood in disarray. Pale flesh and slack muscles hung from diminished bones. Each soft breath moved the sheet so little that I had to look closely to detect the motion.

I inched around to see his face, a face driven deep into my heart through years and decades. There was no anger there, no scorn or praise. The eyes that had watched me turn, one day at a time, into another person were closed. The ears that had heard me cry and sing and laugh rested unhearing. I wanted to brush his hair back with my hand; he'd be concerned about that. Instead, I looked up at the thin green trace progressing across the monitor. Minor detours appeared, subtle changes moved the pace along, but the overall pattern remained consistent.

He stirred. Some hidden dream rose close enough to the surface that he shifted his hips, flexed his jaw, then settled back into the steady dip and beep of postoperative sleep. Was he dreaming about B-17s over Texas? Or cargo planes in the dark skies of the South Pacific? I hoped he was someplace where small kids jumped into his lap, or cold beers foamed bridges between young airmen who leaned laughing against shiny American cars.

My heart assumed that slow rhythm advancing across the screen. For just one second, the small, gray man in the cold steel bed was large and strong again. Dry hospital winds turned warm. Again I missed the baseball he tossed, felt the disappointment, felt the pain, touched the cool green grass of one distant summer. Saw the smile and sparkling blue eyes as he shook his head and clapped his hands for me to throw it back.

Instead, I sank into a cloudy day, where one old sergeant lay sleeping, surrounded by his son and two hearts drawn together across the flickering screen.

He Lifted His Eyes

Nancy Keene

I felt sour nausea rise at my first glimpse of the flowering cherry trees that line the hospital driveway. I had made this trip so many times in the last two years, silent child by my side. That first night, Valentine's Day, 1992, she was a pale, bruised 3-year-old with a white blood cell count of 240,000. Michelle had unfortunately joined the ranks of children with the most common childhood cancer, acute lymphoblastic leukemia.

But today we had a different mission: port removal. Treatment had concluded, medically a rousing success. But the little girl huddled at my side, who didn't talk to most people and still had trouble with balance and sequential thought processes, wasn't feeling so lucky. She was scared.

Weeks before, she had threatened to "slice that thing out of me with a knife." She hated the port. She hated the way it made her chest look, hated the pokes into her breast, hated everything about it. I explained the reasons why it was better to leave it in until treatment was over, but I assured her that the surgeon would give it to her to do with as she wished. She talked of stomping it flat, tying it into knots, and cutting it into small pieces.

I had arranged for us to be the first surgical case of the day to avoid delays that might escalate her fears. As we sat in the waiting room, she wrapped her arms around herself and began to rock. I stroked her back. We were called into our cubicle and she changed into a child-sized flannel gown.

A tall, red-headed doctor walked in. He looked pale, exhausted, and had bags under his eyes. He shook my hand, introduced himself as the anesthesiologist, and mechanically began the series of questions we had heard many times before: Is she allergic to any medications? Has she had anything to eat or drink since midnight? Does she have any loose teeth? His eyes never left his clipboard. Michelle started rocking faster.

He lifted his eyes from his papers, and silently watched the tiny, hunched figure desperately trying to rock her fear away. He said, "Michelle, are you worried?" She remained silent.

Then his eyes met mine and he asked, "Is your daughter worried about having her port accessed this last time?" I thought of saying, "Terrified would be a better term," but I merely replied, "Yes, she is." He looked at Michelle and gently said, "Would you rather have gas, with no pokes? I'll let you pick your favorite flavor." She nodded and stopped rocking. She chose bubble gum.

I explained to him that we wanted to take the port home with us. He said he didn't think it would be a problem. I looked him in the eyes and said, "I promised."

He asked me what Michelle's favorite bedtime story was and I said that she might enjoy *The Three Bears* since she had lately been calling herself a small bear. He let Michelle play with the bubble-gum mask, explained what was going to happen, and promised her the port. He put the mask on her face, leaned down, and whispered, "Once there were three bears: Papa Bear, Mama Bear, and a beautiful small bear named Michelle." She drifted off with a smile on her face.

I found a quiet corner out in the corridor and wept. I wept for all of the tired residents who had been so tender with my fragile child; I wept for her stolen childhood; I wept thinking of the many times I carried her here to be hurt; I wept because I had recently learned that safe sedatives were often used to prevent children's pain and terror during procedures, but they were not offered at our clinic; and I wept with gratitude because she was alive and most probably would grow up, marry, and have her own babies some day.

Then I went into the bathroom, threw cold water on my face as I had done so many times before, and went back to meet her. A nurse brought Michelle out, still asleep but smiling, clutching a Baggie with the bloody port in it.

The next day, I wrote a note to that anesthesiologist, thanking him for not only practicing the mechanics but the art of medicine. He had noticed a little girl's unstated fears and transformed the last, dreaded procedure into a gentle triumph.

Windows

Frank D. Campion

It seems to be getting harder and harder for the layperson to make the necessary, crucial medical decisions only he or she can make. Costs have risen, of course. Ethical questions are more complex. And the growth of scientific technology has made many things more difficult to understand. The voice of common sense, of humane reason, does not come through with the strength we might like.

Not that I have anything against the strides made in medicine. High-tech medicine stood me in good stead in my first brush with laryngeal cancer ten years ago, and it seemed to be doing well in managing a recurrence that appeared last fall. But suddenly, this April, as I struggled to recover from radiation therapy, all of my energy, appetite, and strength seemed to go. A CT scan confirmed the worst suspicion: a new tumor was growing in my neck between the airway and the esophagus. My case had taken on a new, possibly terminal dimension.

At this point I was in the hospital for tests. The results for some of these were still pending, and my surgeons were due for an out-of-town meeting. The preliminary decision to operate had been made, but the difficult first step—chemotherapy—was at least a week away. "Why not go home?" my personal physician suggested.

Even after only a week or so in an excellent hospital, my going home was a great change for the better. Our bedroom looks west, through French doors and organdy curtains into a growth of white spruce, elm, and silver maple. It was a warm, sunny day when I came home. A faint breeze stirred the green boughs outside and carried the distant voices of the cardinal and mourning dove. Then, into this agreeable, innocent setting came a terribly out-of-place thought: what a lovely place to die.

At first it was neither a totally serious nor a totally frivolous thought, but it was one on which I found myself spending more and more time. After discussing my feelings with my physician, he discontinued my mild antianxiety medication temporarily. Both of us wanted my mind clear and uninfluenced. The out-of-place thought started to settle in.

I began to examine the risks and rewards of the proposed surgery, a difficult and complex choice for anyone, let alone a layperson. My physicians were patient and considerate, desirous of making things open and clear. I finally decided that I would be in for a long hospital confinement, prolonged suffering, and results that would barely justify the risks, assuming the surgery was successful in the first place.

Within our family, the most vocal and articulate supporter of the no-surgery decision was my son-in-law. Both of his parents had died after long illnesses, his father from diabetes-related heart disease, his mother from cancer. "A long illness eventually destroys the love between people," he said, "erodes it, just wears it out. That's what happened in our family. I've always felt I never had the chance to say good-bye to either one of my parents. They died in different years, but I think I was the only one in the family to notice they died on the same day of the year."

Once I decided (and I should say that my wife Georgene and four children joined in the decision) to let nature take its course, the relief was enormous. First to go was the three-times-a-day torture at the dining table. For seven-and-a-half months I had been asked "to eat," yet my appetite was nil; swallowing was painful, and thickened saliva made chewing difficult. My wife and I would rack our brains each morning to try to think of something that would "go down" that evening. For both of us each day began with "Oh, God, what will we do about dinner tonight?" Perhaps that doesn't sound like much, but try the mental strain for seven-and-a-half months. About this time I also developed sleep problems. I don't like pills, and I don't usually take them, except under conditions of injury or illness. The sleeping medicines I used were either ineffective or produced nightmares. I was too tired just to put on the light and read, which is what I used to do.

I am now sleeping well and am in no pain. My decision was certainly affected by an illness' eventual ability to cause emotional (as well as physical) death. It also set forth an outpouring of love and feeling among all in our family. It established a new level of love between me and my wife, between brother and sister, between half brother and half sister.

None of this is to downplay high-tech medicine. We need every bit of it we can get. But, it can get in the way of decisions that emphasize the all-important human factor.

Sometimes we let the technology of medicine interfere too much with people who enjoy sunny windows.

Believer

Kathy Swackhamer

It's August in Phoenix, hot as the earth's beginning. I am attending a neuroscience conference. My 8-year-old son, Jay T., is autistic.

The inside of my head is crammed with pharmacology, neuropathology, and epileptology. For three years I have been maneuvering through medical science like a tourist lost in downtown traffic.

Autism is blatantly wrong. It is maladaptive. I know it; Jay T. knows it. He wants out.

"Are you normal yet?" His hands flap in wingbeats below his chin. He toe-steps in place.

"'Am I,'" I correct.

"Am I normal yet?" His high-pitched voice is raspy. Blue eyes probe me with intensity.

"Not when you scream, kick, and bite people," I say

"You want to be normal!" he screeches. Flopping to the floor, he flails his legs in the air. "Normal, normal. This program has also been made possible with financial support of viewers like you. This program has also been made possible by. . . . "

"Stop! No more." I hold my ears and rock slightly, modeling his technique.

I have been interviewing physicians and researchers throughout the world. There is a certain symmetry to their responses. I'd like to break it.

"Jay T. is damaged. I can't help you."

I say nothing, but I want to grab their shoulders and shake them. "Don't give up on us so easily!"

And when the door clicks shut, I whirl around silently, muttering, "All right, we'll do it ourselves."

Autism walks with Jay T. like a shadow, growing and diminishing. Intangible but persistent, it retreats only in the dark as he sleeps.

When he awakens, Jay T. charges out of bed to the stereo where he slips on headphones and listens intently to *Phantom of the Opera*. If the selection on the CD player is anything other than *Phantom,* he shrieks while kicking tables, flipping chairs, and striking out at anyone within reach. Then abruptly he begins to weep, a timeless wailing, unchildlike in its profound grief.

Later he adds and subtracts numbers in his workbooks or obsessively lists the previous day's events. With his uneven motor control, he inscribes letters and numbers hieroglyphic-like on endless pages.

Throughout the day he searches for apostrophes. He locates them on signs, cereal boxes, books.

"Is that an apostrophe?" His body trembles; his eyes are wet with joy.

But his real friends are the newscasters. He tracks their appearance and mourns their absence. For special occasions his conversations with them include Spanish.

"Jane Pauley will be sitting in for Tom Brokaw tomorrow. Tom, are you sick? See you Lunes. See you mañana, Jane Pauley."

His vision of order is sacred. I never dare trespass on it.

I have not counted the trials of medication, the diets, the neurosurgery, the behavioral programs. If they total 500, there are 500 fewer to try.

At the conference I seek information about autism, but research is scarce. Most experts today regard autistic children as irreversibly dysfunctional. The view overlooks Jay T.'s special abilities, such as reading at age 2 or remembering the names of everyone who has ever visited his home with the precise date of the visit. It disregards his uncommon perceptions. When his 3-year-old brother executed an extraordinary temper tantrum, Jay T. observed: "Is the normal one autistic?"

These researchers, like atheists, contend that the curious latencies and flickers of wholeness are illusions. Their plan is to eliminate autism through prevention. They hope to identify defective genes.

Shopping research booths, I locate a study on naltrexone, a drug used for heroin addicts.

"Hi. I'm a parent of an autistic child. Will you explain your findings to me?"

Obligingly, she shares her research. The drug is safe and shows promise. I take several reprints of the study for Jay T.'s physicians. The researcher admonishes: "It may be helpful—not a cure."

I stride out the convention doors into breath-contracting heat. A possibility sits magnified in my brain.

I'm a believer. I believe in apostrophes and hieroglyphics. I also believe in the spirit that moves the pulse in my temples and the unguarded imagination that can make right what matters most to me.

I believe my son can get well. I'm a believer.

Before the examination started, he held the instrument against my thigh and asked if it was warm enough. Something so simple put me in control. When he finished the examination and the nurse left the room, he said, "Everything looks healthy. Anything else I can answer for you?"

"No, but it looks like I picked the right doctor. You're very kind and compassionate."

He looked surprised. But I wasn't.

I now understood why his waiting room was packed. His patients were willing to wait for a doctor who took time to listen, to reassure, to treat each as an individual with a life, not just a patient with a problem. Michael Balint termed this exchange "a mutual investment company." This "company" is based on the premise of listening to help nurture an open and honest relationship between physician and patient, one that can increase in value with each exchange.

I don't know anything about Dr Goodwin's training, but I know he values the art of listening. He used it like a tool throughout the interview. He looked me straight in the eye when talking to me. He asked me three times if he could answer any questions. When I spoke, I knew he was listening carefully. He mirrored back my words and paid attention to my body language. He encouraged me to tell him the truth.

I opened up to him not knowing that I had anything to say. He took my thinking mind and my feeling body into consideration when he spoke. He did something very simple: he accepted me as a whole person.

I don't remember much about his face. In my mind, he is an ageless person with a kind, soothing voice, open ears, and a gentle physical and emotional touch. To me, this is what it means to be a healer.

Thank you, Dr Goodwin, for treating me as a whole person, for remembering my name, for acknowledging my dreams, for "normalizing" my fears, for treating me with compassion. You gave me dignity to leave with confidence, and to return with courage. Thank you for investing in me. Please know that I've invested in you too.

When You Come Into My Room

Stephen A. Schmidt, EdD

When you come into my hospital room, you need to know the facts of my life

that there is information not contained in my hospital chart

that I am 40 years married, with four children and four grandchildren

that I am "genetically Lutheran" . . . with gut disease, like Luther himself

that I am a professor

that I teach teachers, priests, sisters how to nurture faith in the next generation

that I love earthy sensuous life, beauty, travel, eating, drinking J&B scotch, the theater, opera, the Chicago Symphony, movies, all kinds, water skiing, tennis, running, walking, camping

that I love loving, the wonder and awe of sexual intimacy

that I enjoy gardening, smell of soil in misty rain and scorching sun

that I have led a chronic illness group for 12 years

When you come into my room, you need to know the losses of my life

that I have Crohn's disease and three small-bowel resections

that I have been hospitalized more than a dozen times for partial bowel obstruction

that I am chronically ill, and am seeking healing, not cure

that my disease has narrowed my life, constricted it

that I once fantasized but no longer dream about being president of Concordia or Mundelein College that I can no longer eat fresh salads or drink a glass of wine

that I love teaching but sometimes have no energy left at the end of the day

that my Crohn's disease is active in the fall and spring, cyclically in tune with my work

that when I was to give my presidential address to the Association of Professors and Researchers in Religious Education, I was in the hospital for surgery

that when a colleague read my speech, I felt professionally diminished

that I can travel only where there is modern technology . . . I need fiberoptic intubation

When you come into my room, you need to know my body

that I am afraid of medical procedures done at night . . . I awake fearfully to ten feet of air in an IV tube . . . I kink the tube and call . . . nurses come quickly . . . but I will not forget . . . and my body remains sleepless in any hospital

that I know the loss of 25 pounds, not recorded in my chart . . . I had to beg for a subclavian catheter for additional nutrition before I received one

that I am afraid of fifth-year residents . . . they tell me if my intestine does not open in four more days, I will have to have another surgery . . . information not helpful or useful

that I am on Pentasa, prednisone, Bentyl, Questran, vitamin B_{12}, Relafen . . . more than 20 pills each day . . . if I remember

that I hate rounds held outside my room, rounds that do not include nurses, my wife, my children, my pastor, or even me . . . rounds done over me, around me, but not with me

that this body seems battered, old, vulnerable, tired . . . but still me

that I live by medication

that I live by technology

that I live by waiting, in the eternal "advent season" of doctors' offices

When you come into my room, you need to know my heart

that I am emotional . . . a fully functioning feeling person

that I am afraid of the NG tube, sometimes wrapped in my mouth, clogged

that I fear surgery, each time

that I once felt I could not breathe in recovery

that I fear awakening from surgery with an ostomy

that with each partial obstruction I am anxious about another surgery

that I have lost confidence in my body

that I experience sadness and depression more often now than before the
disease

that many persons chronically ill consider suicide, I am one of them

that the advent of symptoms is scary and debilitating

that I am angry at life's unfairness: my brother, older, eats too much
drinks too much plays too much and is healthy, always healthy

so too my wife

and it seems also my colleagues . . . like I once was but am no longer, ever

that I worry about the future . . . insurance

that I am anxious about aging and how I will cope

that I long for one perfect day, only one symptom-free 24 hours

that I lust for remission

that being sick is narcissistic, boring, dull, painful

that there are times I want to give up

**When you come into my room, you need to know my mind and
my spirit**

that I seek meaning in suffering

that suffering is the nudge to the religious question

that I have faith and lose it

that I cling to my faith in spite of all evidence opposite

that I am trapped by the struggle for meaning yet engaged by it

that I am slowly coming to believe that meaning is what we bring to
suffering, not what we gain from it

that God, faith, meaning, ultimate concern, love, salvation are the being of
my being

that I struggle with God

that Job was more just than God

that in my religious quest words are important, music is a mirror to my
soul, and Eucharist, the stuff of mystery

that I believe deeply that I need to engage suffering

that disease forces the God question and nurtures the Godless response

that illness focuses the issue of death

When you come into my room, you need to sustain my hope
You need to know that I believe love wins over hate, hope over despair,
    life over death
that I hope against hope
that I pray and believe prayer heals
that some days I am able to make meaning of suffering
that I am more gentle, more compassionate, better with dying, more
    loving, more sensitive, deeper in grief and in joy

Sit at my "mourning bench" if you are my physician
    listen to me, talk truthfully to me
you need to know all this if you want to heal me

And bear my rage about my disease
that I will never be cured
that my daughter has Crohn's disease and is only 33 years old
that she too has had her first surgery and lives with many of my feelings
and I am angry and sad

And support my hope
that tomorrow there may be new medicines
that today you care deeply
that you will do your best

When you come into my hospital room, promise me presence
promise me a healing partnership
keep hope alive
it is all I have.

The Ear

Lauri Umansky Onek

My child has a birth defect. I hasten to add that it is a mild one, and that it has been corrected in large part by surgery.

But that caveat must not erase the essence of what I have to say.

Her right ear was smaller than the left. It was malformed, turned inward slightly, with two tiny skin tags hanging from it.

The doctors commented on it even as they cleaned her off, as I lay post-cesarean, aching through the middle, hollow with fear.

"The other ear looks fine," they said as they placed the baby in her father's arms.

Then I held her: the sweet damp belly, the eager lips, the reddish ringlets, the ten toes, the clench. And the ear.

"Be grateful," my mother said. "She is beautiful, she is healthy. She is your child. Love her, enjoy her. An ear is a very small part of a life."

As I lay crying for the next two days, specialists came and went from my hospital room, hooking up the baby to machines, reporting with relief and solicitude that her left ear could hear perfectly, that it would compensate for the right, which had no discernible eardrum and was, for all functional purposes, "useless."

The mother of my hospital roommate told me that her son had been born deaf in one ear and that he had never been affected by the shortcoming.

We have seen children so malformed, the nurses told me, that they looked like monsters. Be grateful for what you have.

I am. When I have taken Carenna to the children's hospital for the multiple operations to clear up subsequent complications of the defect, and I have seen the children with heads too large, heads too small, legs twisted, legs absent, hair sparse from chemotherapy, eyes vacant in exaggerated sockets, mobility so limited as to call the definition of living into question. I have known, at the deepest, even cellular level, that all of life is a gift, capricious, precious, momentary.

I understand that my child's birth defect is mild, as such things go. So one ear is a bit smaller than the other. A bit misshapen. After much surgery, my daughter now suffers only a 30% hearing loss in the ear, and that loss has not seemed to have affected her functional hearing in any way. She is a happy, beautiful, dimpled, curly-haired 5-year-old child who belts out the tunes to *The Little Mermaid* with the best of them, who takes on any jungle gym undaunted, who truly believes she is an incarnation of Pippi Longstocking. A normal, spirited child.

I look at Carenna from one angle and say to myself, it is hardly discernible. I look at her from another, and I see the imperfection quite clearly. I fiddle with her hair, never able to cover the ear, because her very curly hair grows out and out, never down. I curse the maternal and paternal genes, silently.

I cry many days about the ear. I wonder what I did wrong during my pregnancy. Was it the photocopy machine? Was it the glass of wine I drank before I knew I was pregnant? On my most difficult days, I wonder if it was the inevitable fate of a child of mine, a reflection of the ineffable wrongness of me.

I feel guilty for indulging this sadness, when indeed the defect is mild. Yet I feel it. Why my child?

It is a cute little ear, really. Not quite formed, it looks fetal, like a curled fern, a glimpse of something sacred. Secretly, I adore the "little ear." I plant kisses around it. It is our miracle ear, once destined never to hear.

It is not that I am ungrateful.

But the ear does not hear fully. And it looks different. And she comes home now from camp with the taunts of the older boys, who bully her into believing that she has no eardrums at all, believing that she is an embodiment of difference and shame. Kids can be ignorant and cruel, we tell her. Everyone has something different about them, some things more obvious than others. Difference can be something positive. We love your ear. It is cute. You have the right to be in the world, however you are, and you have the right to be loved, cherished, and accepted. We love, cherish, and accept you.

"I just want to be normal," she says. "I don't want a magic ear or a cute little ear. I want ears like all the other kids. I don't want them to tease me."

I hold her. She cries and cries. It does not help her to know that there are other children who are worse off, any more than it helps me. Her pain engulfs her. She is only 5. There is so much more to come.

But the next day, she comes to me pertly, having figured it all out.

"Those boys don't make sense. Now, if I had NO eardrums, how could I hear? I have a big ear and a little ear. The big ear hears better. Why do they have such a hard time understanding that?"

"They wonder about themselves," I say.

She nods, sagely.

I hope she will remember that moment of knowing.

I kiss the little ear passionately, and I come incrementally closer to embracing the beleaguered, hungry child that I have always been. The ear *is* little. And it *is* lovable.

Through the Looking Glass

Hester Hill Schnipper, LICSW

Before

As hard as it is to remember, there was a before. I have been an oncology social worker for almost 20 years. I have been a daughter, a sister, a mother, a wife, a lover, a friend. I have been healthy and strong and felt myself to be invulnerable. I have run a marathon to prove to myself that I could meet any challenge. I look now at pictures taken before and try to see a difference, try to understand.

In 1991, in a journal article, I wrote that "for both patients and caregivers, this free-floating awareness of life's end creates a special, shared definition of time which is experienced as having both length and breadth—as well as being sharply divided by 'pre' and 'post' cancer. Both patients and caregivers believe that quality, not only quantity, of life is most important and that the experience of life can be cherished."

We who work for years as caregivers in the field of oncology may learn the lessons our patients have to teach. We know that life is fragile and fleeting, and that we can find no real control and no safety. We know that there is no real boundary between us, and that we must together face the tiger.

We think, or at least I thought, that we know all about it.

Diagnosis

For years, in both my public and private lives, I have said, "When I get breast cancer. . . ." When asked if I had been through the experience, I responded, "Not yet." Did this prescience come from my mild family history or, more likely, from the years of sitting with women who were just like me except that they had already been diagnosed? It is impossible to sustain denial and belief in the power of healthy living when confronted daily by the others.

We who work in oncology may believe at some primitive level that we have struck a bargain with the gods. Even if we deny this belief in our heads, in our hearts the pact has been sealed. We take on seemingly endless loads of sadness; we sit too often with grief. We may think this will buy us and those whom we love protection.

During the fall of 1992, as I neared my 44th birthday, I felt vaguely, diffusely unwell. I was certain that there was something very wrong with me.

On February 8, 1993, early in the morning as I stretched, my fingers went straight to a lump in my breast that had not been there before.

I knew—even though later that day a friend, who is a surgeon, said, "I am not very worried, but the only way to be sure is to biopsy it. Knowing you and what you do, you can't live with the uncertainty." The mammogram that evening, like its decade of annual predecessors, showed nothing.

Then there was the otherworldness of the OR, of straddling the line between patient and caregiver. I went to the biopsy under an assumed name. I changed from suit and silk blouse to johnny and foam slippers in the women's OR locker room. I joked with the surgeon and with the nurses and tried to hold on to my role of "one of us," not "a patient."

During the surgery, my doctor said, "It's out," and left to hand-carry the specimen to Pathology where other friends—pathologist and oncologist—were waiting. She did not return to the OR. Instead, someone said, "Your doctor will talk with you in a few minutes." I knew.

After telling me that I had cancer, my surgeon wept. Then we wept together. And then she promised me that she would not cry into the incision at the next surgery.

Hearing the diagnosis is only the first, and not necessarily the hardest, assault. One also has to tell it to one's partner, to children, to parents, friends, and colleagues. Even harder, the truth has to be integrated into the self. Standing before the mirror, over and over I said the words: "I have cancer."

Hearing the diagnosis brought the longing to be held by him I love the best. In trying to love it away together, in the midst of the loving, we wept. Hearing brought the worst fear I could imagine, the fear of leaving behind motherless children. We acknowledge our shortcomings as parents; we appreciate that we mother or father imperfectly. But we expect to give our children safe passage to adulthood, to shield, protect, nurture, and love them until they can stand alone. Hearing meant I might not live to do so. It meant also telling my mother, herself a breast cancer survivor and a widow to cancer, that her own cry of "What have I done to you?" will echo through another generation. Hearing meant sitting silent and stunned in my office minutes after the diagnosis with my dearest friends and colleagues who shared my world. I knew that their sense of security was utterly shaken as I had suddenly become our mutual worst nightmare.

Hearing meant lying on the winter ground, flattened to the earth. Was I trying to join with the very soil or practice being part of it? It meant stopping by an empty chapel and asking for grace and asking for courage. I was too frightened to ask for cure.

During

The vague pervasive sense of "malaise" that had haunted the previous six months was gone. I moved fugue-like through the stations to which I had accompanied so many others. As they had described, when the pain became unbearable, I too felt my brain shut down, turn off, and self-protectingly declare, "No more."

One of the lessons was learning to say, "Yes, thank you," when help was offered; then, later, discovering that I could even ask for help. Will you come with me for the bone scan? Will you sit, guard and companion, at my bedside the day after surgery? Will you, can you, could you? Each person I asked said yes, and with the collective strength of so many affirmations, I found it possible to go on.

These are lessons new patients learn. However, in my case, I was also thinking about how to care for my own patients. There is little written by social workers or other therapists about how a health professional continues with the work through her own lengthy medical crisis. Does one tell? Whom does one tell? And how?

At the time of my diagnosis, I was leading two breast cancer support groups, one at the hospital and the other in my private practice. The evening private group was a contracted ten-week format; we were at week 7 when I had to cancel a meeting. When we met again, I had decided to say nothing about the cancellation unless someone asked. No one did then or at the remaining sessions, nor did I volunteer any information. My rationale was that these women were paying me to care for them; they needed the space and attention, not me.

The truth was that I could not bear to talk about it.

The second group at the hospital was an ongoing group, and I said nothing for some weeks. But my hair was falling out at an alarming rate; I made my decision and took the plunge. After I told them, there was a profound change in the atmosphere of the therapy. In both group and individual sessions, the almost always unspoken "You can't quite understand because you haven't had it" was gone.

It became clear to me that I needed to be public about my diagnosis; if left unnamed, my cancer would be the charging elephant under the rug. As a result of my disclosure, the quality of my interactions with my patients changed exponentially. The intensity, candor, affect, and opportunities for growth were unparalleled as the work was shared between both of us in the room; the mutual need to search for truth and meaning was remarkable. Even now that I again look healthy and many of my new patients do not know my history, that has stayed true.

Another aspect of the months of treatment was my relationships with colleagues. The experience of my illness frightened everyone; gone were the last hopes of "Cancer can't happen to me." I worried about my friends and my caregivers and was profoundly grateful for their collective attention and affection. I appreciated their honest expressions of concern and learned to depend on their help. I hoped that they all felt, as one of my doctors did, that "I hate taking care of you, but I would hate it worse if anyone else were."

Because of the nature of my work, I was well acquainted with my choices and their risks. I was not frightened by the thought of chemotherapy and was only somewhat bemused by the necessity of lying under a radiation machine. But I was overwhelmed by affect: fear, grief, disbelief, and anger. I found myself bristling with rage and totally at a loss as to how to handle it.

I had opted for a concurrent radiation and chemotherapy protocol and insisted it begin on a particular day so that the radiation would be completed before an important conference that I needed to attend. On the designated day, first my surgeon and then my oncologist examined me. They left the room and conferred in the hall before examining me again. They then left again and were gone a long time before my oncologist returned alone to tell me that she could not begin: My surgical healing was not complete. I was wild with anger and frustration. My life was out of control.

Nothing could be planned. Nothing could be managed. No one cared about me or what was important to me. I raged.

The following Monday, chemotherapy did begin. Although not frightened, I was having difficulty perceiving these powerful drugs as life-giving rather than as poisons. Mostly, I was heartsick as I turned on my Walkman, began the Bach, meditated, and extended my bare arm to my old friend, now my chemotherapy nurse. Instead of finding peace, I found myself seeing in my mind's eye my daughters grow, and I wept. I wept, of course, for all the "Will I live to see . . . ?"

Cancer treatment has a way of emphasizing the physical. I struggled with my body, endured fatigue, radiation burns, chronic nausea, and often worse, knelt each morning on the bathroom floor to sweep up the hair. I felt sick every day for six months.

After

Six days after I took the final Cytoxan pills, my family and I brought home a puppy. As I watched him in my daughter's arms, I wondered which of us would survive the other. I hoped he would be a comfort to her if I died. He is now 90 pounds of healthy creature, and I love him beyond all proper proportions for a dog. He is my commitment to a future and represents my hope.

We know about issues common to cancer survivors. The first and most important is "Am I a survivor? Will I survive this?" We understand that everyone is living on borrowed time, but we live that knowledge. It is not like "Maybe I will be hit by a truck tomorrow." It is intermittent, usually unexpected, paroxysms of feelings that can quite literally take your breath away. Sometimes the fear is like a wildcat on our backs, claws digging in.

Six months after completing chemotherapy, I returned to my surgeon for a routine visit. As she was examining me, her face and body stiffened; she had found a new lump. Again, I entered the OR, endured another biopsy, and finally went home. It was a Friday afternoon, and, so soon after my treatments, I had no reserves, no coping capacity. I spent the weekend under the quilts, napping and reading and hiding. On Monday morning, my doctor told me that all, this time, was well.

My work life continues. I answer my phone to hear a patient/friend weeping; she is at her surgeon's office and has been told that her breast cancer has spread to her brain. I sit with a patient/friend whose initial presentation was very much like my own; she now has widely metastatic disease. I accompany a patient/friend to her initial consultation with the bone marrow transplant team. I sit with a dying woman and her daughter, who is exactly the same age as my younger girl; we talk and plan together for this girl's life after her mother's death. My brain and my heart are exploding; I want to cradle my body and rock, to scream and to weep. How can I possibly help this woman when I am so overwhelmed by my own fear and grief? How can I not when helping her means helping me? It is the best way I can fight back.

As months pass, I have become more comfortable in my skin; I again fit my clothes, run most mornings, and brush a full head of hair. I try to trust my body. Always there are parallel tracks of hope and planning inside me; each decision must be marked by a two-angle lens: the maybe-I-will-live-for-years view and the maybe-I-will-die-soon one. Every goal, plan, thought, and relationship must be forced through a double filter.

I am part of an astonishing collection of women. I am so proud of my sisters as we, alone and together, live with breast cancer. I give thanks for my companions on this journey.

I have found courage. I have been given grace. I love my life.

The Venetian Blinds

Lee Litvinas

The morning sun filtered through the venetian blinds, casting dancing columns of light on the wall beside my hospital bed. Today will be the day. No more suffering for my family and myself. No more sleepless, sweatful, painful nights. Life will go on for the masses, struggling with the meaning of their existence. Today, I, like others before me, will experience the truth and freedom that only death can bring. Yes, today is the day. The doctors have played all their cards. They have worked their pseudo-miracles, filling me with toxins, technology, and nausea.

Safe, uneventful passage is all I desire, and yet this is precisely what is denied me. I have no appetite, yet I am fed through my veins. I have lost inspiration, yet I receive manufactured air through a hot, oily machine. So foreign now are the pictures coming from the television suspended near the ceiling of my room. I am no longer of this world. How long must I endure this meaningless, helpless existence in which strangers are salaried to care for me day in and day out, removing the feces from my bed? My nakedness is but a trivial consideration for my caretakers. I have lost all individuality. I have been reduced to a data-generating organism, verifying the laws of physiology.

Oh, today will be the day, today must be the day of my liberation.

"Good morning, Mr Olson," spoke the young doctor, medical chart in hand, as he entered my room. "The nurses tell me you are doing quite well today. Your vital signs couldn't look better, and your blood tests are even more encouraging. I must say, you are rapidly becoming one of our success stories around here. Why, I think that in a week or two we'll have you out of the intensive care unit and to a regular room. Of course, you know that you will need the respirator indefinitely, but then that's not so bad, it could be a lot worse, you know."

No, it couldn't be any worse than the present, and there was no time like the present.

"Let me loosen your wrist restraints so I can examine you and get a closer look at you," said the doctor as he untied my wrist from the bed rail. He needed to verify the laws of physiology for himself. If I could just gather my strength I might have a chance. Yes, today is the day! My heart began to pound, each beat flushing my face with a wave of heat and desperation. The doctor placed his stethoscope on my naked chest. His eyes studied my face with scientific objectivity. I saw my frightful, wasted features in the reflection of his wire-rimmed glasses. Tears began to well up in my eyes. My hands clenched into fists as my arms tensed. Liberation was at hand. My arm was in motion with a powerful swing, landing my knuckles squarely in the reflection of those wire-rimmed glasses. The doctor fell back, staggering, with an outstretched arm to brace his fall. His glasses shattered against the wall behind him. Now the respirator, the final act of destiny, the tube in my throat must go! With the same powerful swing of freedom I grasped and pulled. I was extubated and breathless. My thoughts began to spin. Then there were no thoughts, no sounds, only a sense of floating, drifting above my hospital bed and seeing myself lying amidst the timeless chaos of the event.

But slowly my etherealness began to fade and my drifting became weighted. I could hear the voices of the doctors and nurses surrounding my bed. I could feel my wrist restraints once again. The hot respirator air was expanding my chest. My escape had been foiled.

"Ten milligrams of Valium, stat!" shouted a doctor. "This guy needs some sleepers!"

And then there was nothingness until morning. The breathing machine moaned on. I had returned to my cage of earthly consciousness. The shadows of the venetian blinds were cast across my bed as though bars around a desperate criminal.

Come Follow Me

Louis M. Profeta

Come—follow me. Today I am going to walk you through the third floor of the Children's Pavilion. Before we go upstairs, let's sit down and imagine we are young again. Think about the neighborhood playground; see yourself playing kickball, climbing the jungle gym, jumping rope. If you listen, you can hear the laughing, the playful screams of childhood. Close your eyes and think about how strong and indestructible you are as a child, how carefree. There are no such things as cancer, pneumonia, muscular dystrophy, spinal meningitis. There are only youth, happiness, and health. Let's go upstairs.

This is the spinal recovery ward of the pavilion. Nowhere in the world are you as close to the outdoors and yet as far away. There are patients on this ward who have not been outside of the hospital for a year. The third floor is a sea of lifeless limbs and painted smiles. There is not much hope or expectation here. There are no promises or guarantees. You are probably wondering what you have to do to get placed on this ward. The answer is simple: you have to live.

As we walk through this ward, you can see the similarities in each room. All televisions are turned to the afternoon cartoons. Coyote chases Roadrunner, but ends up falling off a cliff and onto his head. If you look carefully, you can see each child flash an uncomfortable grin. Coyote is going to end up here if he's not careful. Mom is sitting in the chair in the corner, reading a Gothic novel or a magazine. She has been here since 9 this morning, just as she is every day. At 12 she will help the nurse feed her son. Don't misunderstand me. This ward is not plain and unexciting; there is variety.

At 1 o'clock the afternoon movie comes on. Mom puts her book down, picks up her knitting, and works on a sleeve. In the end, every sweater is four or five sizes too big. She might put her work aside for a moment, ask her son if he wants a soft drink, walk down the hall, and gaze out the window. She'll let her mind wander for a moment, remember why she is here, and return to the room and again ask if he wants a drink. At 2, the mail arrives. There are usually three or four get-well-soon cards. They have been arriving for seven months now.

The movie is over at 3, and since there is usually nothing on television at that time, the patient calls the nurse for his pain shot. While Mom looks on, the nurse pulls back the covers to reveal a once healthy, robust frame reduced to nothing. Through narrowed eyes, Mom watches the nurse lift a large syringe to the sky. Framed against soft light, a thin stream of morphine arcs through the air and falls gently downward.

During the next two hours Mom will read each card on the corkboard twice. She will stroll down to the nurses' station and talk about the patient in room 303, who fell while on the trampoline. It seems that he was once a nationally ranked gymnast. It is hard to feel sorry for someone else's child when your own son is completely paralyzed. It's time for her to return to her son's room. He will be waking soon and she wants to be there when he does. For the next half hour she will sit and listen to the hospital sounds.

There is so much loud silence on this floor. Her son's graveled breathing is hypnotizing. She can almost imagine his lungs filled with broken glass, as pneumonia finds itself a home. Down the hall she can hear a steady, dull pattering as a therapist drums a beat on a child's back, hoping to break up congestion. At the nurses' station, ECGs harmonize to the sounds of paging, while hurried footsteps grace the corridor.

The room is peacefully disguised. Flowers line the radiator, carnations, mums, a rose, some lilacs from the neighbor's bush. A couple friends sent some of those aluminum-looking helium balloons. All the air has seeped out, and they now hang limp and lifeless on the closet door. On the cart sits an assortment of Martha Washington chocolates. Naturally, a few of the coconut creams remain. Someone brought a stuffed bear and a Rubik's cube; she really can't remember who. On a hook in front of a Steele landscape hangs an IV. She traces the path of the tubing from the ceiling to her son's withered wrist. The air has a strange smell of lilacs, alcohol, and dying.

Every room on this floor is like every other, a series of endless mirrors. Each scene repeats itself over and over again to a private audience, which has paid an exorbitant price to be here. If you look at this room, you will see that this patient is waking up, getting ready for the afternoon scenario. Mom is busy straightening up the room for visitors, who will soon be stopping by to see how everything is going. In about 15 minutes Dad will be arriving from work and will want to speak with Mom and the doctor. It won't really do any good, but this is a ritual that each father must go through. You see, Dad is supposed to take care of his family. If he had been doing his job, none of this would have ever happened.

There is about ten minutes left before family and friends start to arrive to offer their support and prayers. This allows Mom and Dad just enough time to sit in the lounge, drink a cup of coffee, and discuss how to file the insurance claims. This is the parents' lounge, well stocked with tissues and coffee. This is where misery goes to find a family. On the couch lies one of the many fathers, fast asleep and dreaming about the day they called him from work to come to the hospital. His daughter dove into a shallow pool. In his mind, she has been locked into that frame for years. First there were the tongs. He can still see the doctors drilling the bolts into her head, her eyes wide open and aware. He can even hear the crackling as the pins pierced her skull. The screams were deafening. The doctors say she took the pain extraordinarily well. He is awake now.

Visiting hours have started. They are usually signaled by an "Oh, look who's here." Up and down the hall, there is the same sound, "Oh, look who's here." "Say 'thank you.'" "Aunt Jane brought you some Martha Washington chocolates." "He's doing fine. He's been sleeping most of the afternoon." "The doctor says she is doing very well." "Going home in a few weeks." "Going home in a month." "They have not told us very much." In a few moments visiting hours will be over. There will be a couple more cards on the corkboard, another issue of *Sports Illustrated* on the cart, a few more mums and maybe even a spider plant.

It's getting late and our tour is about over. In every room Mom and Dad are kissing their sons and daughters good night. Familiar phrases can be heard above the whirr of respirators. "I'll be back in the morning." "Do you need anything?" "I'll call you when I get home." "I love you." "Take care of yourself." "Get some rest." "Are you sure you don't want me to stay the night?" "Good night."

This is the third floor of the Children's Pavilion. Is it what you expected? We didn't see some Santa passing out toys, a magician entertaining the ill. We saw only parents. We did not even talk to a patient. But for now we must let these people get some rest. It is getting late and there is nothing on television worth watching anymore. In each room a nurse lifts a large syringe to the sky. Framed against the soft light a thin stream of morphine arcs through the air and falls. See you tomorrow at 9.

Long Ago Today

Joseph J. Gallo, MD

It was such a simple thing, merely a touch of the hand. Others had touched her also, but their touch had always seemed so mechanical, so cold, not even fully human. Theirs was a touch of necessity, but this one was different. This was a touch of love, of caring, of humanity. This was a touch that spoke without words, that said, "I know you are a person with a rich history, and not a faceless case or number." This touch allowed her, if only for a moment, to transcend time.

The memories were a hodgepodge of feelings, sights, sounds, and smells, in random order, the way thoughts sometimes run from one to another, connected in peculiar ways. She really couldn't be sure which wisps and glimpses were accurate and which had become enriched with time, but she supposed that didn't matter now.

He had a way of touching her that made her feel secure, his hand firmly wrapped around hers. He was her first and only love. He came so suddenly into her life, accidentally really. She had gone to the dance reluctantly, with her sister. The "boys," as they were called then, were back from Europe. While her sister mingled with the crowd, she receded into the shadows to listen to the band. He was shy too, but managed to strike up a conversation. As one of the "boys," he really hadn't seen much action—the fate of the nations had been sealed—but his experiences seemed to exhilarate and engage her. She didn't remember exactly what was said, but there would be many other nights of long conversations. It was the "feeling" and the atmosphere of the place she recalled best.

He was so proud of their first home. At the time, it didn't seem possible they would ever outgrow it. She remembered he was happy to spend lazy fall afternoons tinkering in the garage. She remembered the cheerful, excited voices of the children playing their simple games. She remembered the smell of freshly baked bread. There is nothing like the aroma of fresh bread, or the buttered taste of it while it's still hot! Over the years the house began to embody family life for her—its nooks, creaks, and furnishings imbued with meaning. Now only a few cherished tokens remain. The things that had seemed so important then now were just hazy memories, faded by time. Still, she was grateful: "One third of a nation ill-nourished, ill-clad, ill-housed" never applied to them.

Her sister calls out—no, she only thinks it's her sister. These days she is distracted easily. It has been a long time since she thought of her sister. She's been long gone. Has it really been 40 years? She can remember glimpses of her as if it were yesterday. Why, she can almost hear her voice, her laughter. And could she dance! Her embrace the night of the wedding was heartfelt and warm, so full of sisterly love. Life was full of promise then.

The emotions rose up inside her. Heaven knows the thinking side, the intellectual side, didn't always seem to work right anymore, but her emotions remained active, vibrant, alive. Even the events of the night her twins were born aren't quite clear anymore, but she remembered well the surge of adrenaline she felt when the time came to have the babies. And how her heart filled with sorrow when she learned one twin died on a faraway beach in a battle they said would change the face of the world. To her it seemed only that it was her face the battle had changed. It wasn't supposed to happen that way.

She sometimes called out to her own mother (or for the comfort and warmth she felt when she thought of her mother). She felt her mother's comforting touch even across the compressed years. Her mother's smile, too, comes back clearly. Mother was preserved as a young woman in her daughter's memory, since she did not share her daughter's good fortune of growing old. And yet, who really was the fortunate one?

It was such a simple thing, merely a touch of the hand, a touch of love, of caring, of humanity. This was a touch that spoke without words, that said, "I know you are a person with a rich history, and not a faceless case or number." She could never express what it had meant, how much she had needed that simple act of human communication.

She so often had felt abandoned in this nursing home. If only daily life were not so devoid of meaning here, even this place could be bearable. There was so much she wished she could share, a lifetime of experiences she needed to come to grips with, to make some sense of life, her life. Wasn't it remarkable how the gentle touch of her doctor reminded her of a time when her life had meaning?

No Better or Wiser, Just Braver and Sicker

Nina Herrmann

I have seen the Fates stamp like a camel in the dark; those they touch they kill, and those they miss live on to grow old.

The Seven Odes

It happened four times in ten days in one children's hospital a winter or so ago. It usually doesn't. Not four times in ten days in one hospital. A pediatric neurosurgeon—a human being—had to walk into four different hospital rooms and face the parents of four different children—also human beings—and say:

"I'm sorry, your child has an inoperable, malignant brain tumor."

"I'm sorry, your child has an inoperable, malignant brain tumor."

"I'm sorry, your child has an inoperable, malignant brain tumor."

"I'm sorry, your child has an inoperable, malignant brain tumor."

Four times in ten days. Four families for whom, from the instant those words were spoken, nothing would ever be the same again.

I have been a hospital chaplain for 20 years. Each day that I've worked at my profession, it has been with children and adults who are dying or are critically ill or have severe and often permanent physical disabilities. Twenty years of it.

I must be nuts.

My reflection on that unsettling fact recently led me to an even more sobering thought: What have I learned in those 20 years as a hospital minister?

Practically, I have learned a lot.

I can describe a VP shunt and some symptoms that can signal its malfunction.

I can list the names of at least eight brain tumors.

I know the side effects of radiation therapy and am learning those of chemotherapy.

I know when observing surgery that I should stand far enough away from the operating table that if I faint forward I won't disrupt anything.

And I can spell myelomeningocele. Not.

But as for how to be a better hospital chaplain and help my patients and families in crisis faith issues, I haven't learned a new thing in 20 years.

In the beginning, I prayed, I stayed, I touched, I hoped; I hurt, I cried, I admitted anger toward God; I hoped and prayed and hoped again. And I went on. Today I pray, I stay, I touch, I hope; I hurt, I cry, I admit anger toward God; I hope and pray and hope again. And I go on.

I would like to tell you something wonderful. I would prefer being able to deliver great words of wisdom gleaned from 20 years of facing disaster and disablement. But from me, there are none. One just goes on or one doesn't.

There *is* one thing I can tell you. But it isn't inspirational. It isn't uplifting. It is simply real. There is one thing that I have learned from experience: the *horror* of knowing what is coming once the words are spoken.

The words can describe a variety of devastating diagnoses, but once spoken, they become as a metronome forever beating, encased in a frozen moment in time:

"I'm sorry, your child has an inoperable, malignant brain tumor."

"I'm sorry, your *child . . .*"

"I'm sorry, *your* child . . ."

"*I'm sorry,* your child . . ."

Then I come in. The minister, the reverend person. Or, at times I am there at the moment, sitting beside the neurosurgeon who must deliver the words. I cannot fathom how the neurosurgeon feels.

But now, after 20 years, I have learned how I will feel. I will feel sick. I will feel sick not only in the depth of my religious being; but I will feel sick in the pit of my human stomach. And a part of me will retain each sick, no matter what else I may be doing.

So I the chaplain sit there in this little hospital conference room and I look at these parents and I feel the horror of knowing what is coming for them and I feel sick. Sick at knowing what the words are. Sick at knowing that their child will become seriously ill and, with statistically few exceptions, will die. And sick at knowing how very, very, very, very long these parents will exist living in shock.

While they are existing living in shock these parents will say and do and think good things and painful things, ordinary things and extraordinary things. They will express angers and hopes. And they will experience fears and guilts and despairs. And they will pray all manner of prayers.

But it will all be done in an environment of shock.

And by the time these parents come out of their shock, they likely will have buried their child.

Shock takes over from the frozen moment the words are spoken until after the child is buried—or cured. And if these parents were *not* in a measurable degree of shock all that time *they would not survive.*

You cannot *sanely* watch your child die. You simply *cannot.* And shock is that which protects us from insanity in the face of the totally irrational.

But shock develops cracks in it here and there along the way to crumbling. And I hospital chaplain have spent 20 years as a guide, waiting and watching for the cracks in the shock. Not to fill them with mortar, for shock *must* crack for healing to begin. But to be there, to be available as one receptacle for that which falls out of the cracks, and as a guide who is about faith.

After 20 years I will go more bravely into the hospital room after the words have been spoken, to lay foundation slowly for when the cracks come. I will pray with, because I know prayer fortifies and gives outlet. I will listen to, because I know that listening is action. I will be with, because I have seen the aloneness wrought by the words. I will touch, because we are human flesh. I will hold, because in the cracking and crumbling of shock I am hospital chaplain trying to represent God who just never stops and leaves *anyone* unheld.

The challenge for me, the challenge after 20 years, is to feel the horror of knowing what lies ahead for these families and still want to. Still want to pray, to listen, to be with, to touch, and to hold.

And I do, still want to. Because, despite all of it and despite not understanding the "Why?" of any of it, I still have hope.

I hope for a cure. A cure from research—*research is vital*—or a cure from a miracle. I always hope and pray for a cure.

I hope for no pain.

I hope for a long remission.

I hope for family survival as a family.

And I hope that the someday crumbling of shock will leave a faith that can make the ultimate difference, enabling these families to go on knowing that despite everything they are held and upheld by God—forevermore.

Is the little 5-year-old boy dead now? He wasn't when I wrote this. The little 5-year-old boy who was one of the four children diagnosed with an inoperable, malignant brain tumor in that ten-day period a year or so ago. He loves Teenaged Mutant Ninja Turtles and pizza with lots of cheese and baseball.

He is an only son.

One winter day I came to the little boy's hospital room to say good-bye before going on a leave. His father was there alone—the little boy was having therapy somewhere else in the building. The lights were dim. I was almost beside this father of an only son before he heard me.

The frozen picture of this man lives glued inside my sick. His head was bent. His hands were fists around a rosary. His lips were moving in step with the repetition of ages. On his face: Tenacious hope . . . behind which the very foundation of all he has ever known of faith begins to tremble.

The hairline crack in the shock had come.

Perspective Shift

Daniel Shapiro, PhD

He looks so sad, so forlorn. He chews a lip as he studies his sneakers. His hands clasp together and then awkwardly separate like uncomfortable acquaintances. His foot drums to a beat internal and irregular. His forehead sweats. The pen in his hand has been chewed and gnawed. Little tooth rivulets carpet its plastic veneer.

I have seen this clinical presentation a thousand times.

The helplessness has surfaced. He can no longer suppress it. He is a steam whistle and the anxiety at facing cancer's horrible ambiguity has finally rumbled to the surface, erupting with volcanic emotional chaos.

He expected better news.

We are staring at chest films that tell a sobering story. A tumor sits in the middle of the chest. An eight-centimeter mass. East to west it is smaller than it was the last time a scan was taken. North to south it appears longer. We both know that nodular sclerosing Hodgkin tumors can leave behind scar tissue. No one can tell if the tumor on this film is alive with cancerous intent or if what we see is a ghostly image of a beast now dead. The oracle of science, on this dry, cold winter day, is silent.

He paces slowly around the large windowed office, lost in thought, unable to find the words to describe his frustration with the unknown. It is painful to watch. These monthly scans have been challenging for him—they've provided so little evidence of progress to encourage the continued fight. Where will the energy come from for more aggressive chemotherapy? More nausea and fatigue? More restless nights?

He is young. He has had little experience with events not in his control. He was brought up on simple just-world ethics. Phrases like "what goes around comes around" pepper his speech and he is always telling me to go see the latest movie portraying a hero surmounting all odds. In his world, good people pull themselves out of poverty and despair and bad ones inevitably pay back in blood for every ridiculing utterance, every nip of ego they've displayed. He cannot reconcile his goodness with today's misfortunes.

I remain silent. He needs to learn to live with the ambiguity. To live, despite the ambiguity. He must come to these understandings on his own. I cannot show him the way. Nor will I offer false hope to make us feel better in this fleeting moment.

Of course I'll be here for him. It's the least I can do. After all, I need him. He is my young doctor and that is my tumor taunting us from the scan.

Glossary

ACE inhibitor   Abbreviation for angiotensin-converting enzyme inhibitor. A class of drugs used in the treatment of **hypertension**.

acetone   A substance produced in very small amounts in normal urine but that can occur in excessive amounts in the urine and blood of persons with **diabetic acidosis**.

acidotic   Increased acid content in the blood and other body fluids that can occur with kidney disease, diabetes, and some diseases of the lungs.

acute lymphoblastic leukemia   Acute lymphocytic leukemia.

acute lymphocytic leukemia   A blood disease characterized by a severe abnormal increase in the number of certain types of white blood cells.

adduction   The movement of a body part toward the midline of the body.

ADLs   Abbreviation for activities of daily living. Routine daily activities (eg, self-care or grooming) that are performed by healthy people.

adrenaline   A hormone (or the drug epinephrine) that helps the body cope with exertion or stress by increasing heart rate and blood flow and improving breathing.

advance directives   Documents, such as a living will or durable power of attorney, that state a person's preferences for end-of-life care.

agonal   Related to the process of dying or the moment of death (eg, agonal breathing).

AIDS   Abbreviation for acquired immunodeficiency syndrome. A fatal disease caused by transmission of **HIV** by way of contaminated body fluids, most commonly semen or blood or blood products. The virus attacks the body's immune system, leaving it defenseless against infection.

air hunger   Deep and labored breathing, or an episode of difficult breathing.

amniocentesis   Insertion of a hollow needle through the abdominal wall and into the uterus to obtain **amniotic fluid** from the amniotic sac. The fluid is then analyzed and can be used to determine abnormalities in or the sex of a fetus.

amniotic fluid   Fluid contained in the amniotic sac that surrounds and protects the fetus during pregnancy.

angina   Chest pain caused by an insufficient supply of oxygen to the heart.

angiocath   Shorthand for angiocatheter. A hollow, flexible tube inserted into a blood vessel and used to administer fluids or drugs.

angiography   A diagnostic procedure that involves injection of a contrast material (special dye) and use of x-rays to visualize the inside of blood vessels.

ankylosing spondylitis   Arthritis (an inflammatory disease) affecting joints in the spine.

anoxic hangover   Jargon for the aftereffects of severe oxygen deficiency.

antigen   A substance capable of inducing an immune response.

antihypertensive   A drug used to reduce blood pressure in persons with **hypertension**.

Apgars   Shorthand for Apgar scores. A rating system used to evaluate the physical condition of a newborn by assigning a value (of 0, 1, or 2) to five criteria (ie, heart rate, respiratory effort, muscle tone, response to stimulation, and skin color).

aphasia   A defect in or loss of comprehension or production of speech or writing due to injury or disease of the brain.

arrest   Shorthand for cardiac arrest. A sudden cessation in the heart's function.

ascites   The accumulation of fluid in the peritoneal cavity (ie, spaces between the tissues and organs in the abdominal cavity).

asystole   The absence of contractions of the heart.

atherogenesis   The formation of fatty deposits on the inner layer of the arterial walls.

atherosclerosis   A disease in which lipid (fat) deposits form on the inner lining of the arterial wall.

attending   Shorthand for attending physician. The staff physician who directs all aspects of a patient's care throughout a hospital stay.

auscultate   To listen, usually with a stethoscope, for sounds within the body, especially in the lungs, heart, and abdomen.

autism   A mental disorder characterized by extreme withdrawal and an inability to relate to people.

axilla   The armpit.

BCG   Abbreviation for Bacille Calmette-Guérin. BCG vaccine is used to prevent tuberculosis and, rarely, is used in cancer therapy.

Bentyl   Trade name for an antispasmodic drug.

Betadine   Trade name for an anti-infective drug applied to the skin.

Biophysical Profile   A numerical scoring system used to assess a fetus in a high-risk pregnancy.

bipolar disorder   A psychiatric disorder characterized by periods of inappropriate euphoria and hyperactivity (mania) and severe depression. Formerly called manic-depression or manic-depressive disorder.

blood gas   Laboratory test that measures the concentration and pressure of oxygen and carbon dioxide in the blood.

bolus   A large and rapidly given injection or ingestion of medication or fluid.

brittle   Unpredictable or unstable (condition of a patient). Often used to refer to patients with diabetes who have wide fluctuations in their blood glucose (sugar) levels.

broad-spectrum   Effective over a wide range. Broad-spectrum antibiotics are effective against more than one type of bacteria.

bronchiectasis   A disorder in which the walls of the air passages in the lungs are stretched and damaged.

BUN   Abbreviation for blood urea nitrogen. A waste product in the blood that is cleared by the kidneys and is measured to determine kidney function.

cachectic   Affected by or relating to a general wasting of the body, due to weight loss, muscle wasting, or both. Usually associated with a long illness or chronic disease.

CAD   Abbreviation for coronary artery disease.

calling it   Jargon for ending a **code**.

cannula   A thin, flexible tube used to introduce fluid into or withdraw fluid from the body.

cardiomyopathy   Disease involving the heart muscle.

cardioversion   Restoring a normal heart rhythm with electric shock to the heart (from a device called a defibrillator).

cathed   Jargon for inserted a **catheter**.

catheter   A thin, hollow, flexible tube inserted into a blood vessel or a body cavity for injection or withdrawal of fluids or to keep a passage open.

CCU   Abbreviation for cardiac care unit or coronary care unit.

cervical intraepithelial neoplasia   Possibly precancerous abnormalities in the cells of the cervix.

chemotherapy   The treatment or control of a disease with chemical medications or drugs; usually refers to cancer treatment.

CHF   Abbreviation for congestive heart failure.

chlamydia   An organism that causes infections, including a common sexually transmitted disease.

chocolate agar   A brown culture medium.

cholecystectomy   Surgical removal of the gallbladder.

cholelithiasis   The formation of gallstones in the gallbladder or bile ducts.

chorea   A disorder of the nervous system characterized by spasms of the limbs and facial muscles and by incoordination.

chylomicron   A type of lipoprotein (a small fat molecule contained in blood).

cirrhosis   A disease that results in scarring of liver tissue and impaired liver function; most commonly due to alcoholism.

CME   Abbreviation for continuing medical education.

CMV   Abbreviation for cytomegalovirus. A type of virus that can cause serious illness in people with weakened immune systems, such as people with **AIDS**.

CNS   Abbreviation for central nervous system (which refers to the brain and spinal cord).

code   A sudden, life-threatening medical emergency involving cardiac **arrest**. Also the medical staff's efforts to restore heart function and breathing.

colostomy   Surgical creation of an artificial opening between the colon and the surface of the body.

compartment syndrome   Compartmental syndrome. A condition in which increased pressure on muscle tissue results in decreased blood flow. Symptoms commonly include muscle weakness, pain, and loss of sensation in the affected area.

coryza   Nasal mucous and discharge resulting from inflammation of the lining of the nasal passage.

CPR   Abbreviation for cardiopulmonary resuscitation. Performing external heart massage and breathing air into the lungs of a person who has no pulse and who has stopped breathing.

crashed   Jargon for a sudden and life-threatening decline in a seriously ill patient.

creatinine   A waste product filtered by the kidneys and excreted in the urine; measured to determine kidney function.

Crohn's disease   A chronic disease characterized by ulcerations in the **gastrointestinal** tract and by narrowing and thickening of the bowel by scar tissue. Symptoms include fever, diarrhea, cramping abdominal pain, and weight loss.

cryptococcal   Relating to or infected by a yeastlike fungus.

C-section   Shorthand for cesarean section (cesarean delivery). A surgical procedure to deliver a baby from the uterus through an incision in the woman's abdomen.

CT scan   Abbreviation for computed tomography scan. A diagnostic imaging technique using special x-rays that produces cross-sectional images of body structures.

cyanosis   Bluish coloration of the skin and mucous membranes caused by an oxygen deficiency in the blood.

cysto   Jargon for cystogram or cystoscopy. Diagnostic studies of the bladder performed by filling the bladder with x-ray dye and taking x-ray films (cystogram) or by examining the inside of the bladder using a special endoscope (cystoscopy).

Cytoxan   Trade name for an anticancer drug.

DCF   DCFS. Abbreviation for Department of Children and Family Services.

defibrillation   Administration of an electric shock to the heart (from a device called a defibrillator) to correct a severely abnormal heart rhythm.

diabetes mellitus   A metabolic disorder, characterized by increased blood glucose (sugar) levels, which results from the body's inability to produce adequate amounts of insulin.

diabetic acidosis   Shift in the acid-alkaline balance of the body to more acidity. Usually associated with uncontrolled **diabetes mellitus**.

diabetic ketoacidosis   Diabetic acidosis.

dialysis   A procedure for removing toxic substances in the blood, most commonly used to treat patients with kidney failure.

diazepam   A drug used as an antianxiety agent, muscle relaxant, and anticonvulsant.

DIC   Abbreviation for **disseminated intravascular coagulation**.

digital replant   Reattachment of a finger or toe after amputation caused by injury.

disseminated intravascular coagulation   A serious condition causing abnormal bleeding in which the body consumes all of its blood-clotting factors. Commonly due to an overwhelming infection.

diuresis   Increased production and excretion of urine.

diverticulitis   Inflammation of the small sacs of the intestinal wall. Symptoms commonly include fever, pain, and tenderness.

DNR   Abbreviation for do not resuscitate.

dobutamine   A drug used to help improve heart pumping function.

dopamine   A drug used to treat very low blood pressure.

DVT   Abbreviation for deep vein thrombosis. Blood clots in the deep veins, usually in the legs or the pelvis.

ecchymotic   Relating to a small, nonelevated red or purplish spot in the skin. Ecchymosis is caused by the presence of blood from ruptured blood vessels into the tissue under the skin.

ECG Abbreviation for electrocardiogram. The curve traced by a machine (an electrocardiograph) used to record heart activity and to help diagnose heart disease.

ECHO Shorthand for echocardiogram. Images of heart structures obtained by using ultrasound. Most commonly used to diagnose heart disease involving the heart valves.

ED Abbreviation for emergency department.

edema Swelling of tissues caused by accumulation of excess fluid, usually involving the lower legs and ankles.

edentulous Having no teeth.

ejection fraction A measurement of ventricular (heart chamber) function.

Elavil Trade name for an antidepressant drug.

electroencephalogram A tracing (made by a machine) that indicates the brain's electrical activity.

electrolytes A group of certain chemicals (eg, sodium or potassium) in the blood.

emesis Vomiting.

emphysema A disease that damages the lungs' air sacs and causes abnormal enlargement of the air spaces. Symptoms commonly include shortness of breath and possibly respiratory or heart failure.

EMT Abbreviation for emergency medical technician.

endometriosis A disorder in which tissue that normally lines the uterus is found in other parts of the pelvis.

endotracheal tube Tube inserted through the mouth or nose into the trachea (windpipe) and used to maintain breathing.

epi Shorthand for epinephrine (**adrenaline**). A drug used to increase heart rate and blood flow.

epicardium Inner layer of the fibrous-serum sac (pericardium) in direct contact with the heart's surface.

epiglottitis Serious condition characterized by inflammation (usually infection) of the flap of thin cartilage tissue (epiglottis) at the base of the tongue. The epiglottis folds over the trachea (windpipe) during swallowing and prevents fluid from entering it.

epileptology The study, diagnosis, and treatment of epilepsy.

ER Abbreviation for emergency room (the emergency department).

erythematous Characterized by skin redness.

erythroblastosis fetalis   A severe disease that is characterized by damage to the red blood cells of a fetus or newborn and leads to anemia, **edema**, and enlargement of the liver and spleen.

erythrophagocytosis   A disorder characterized by ingestion and digestion of red blood cells by other cells known as phagocytes.

esophageal   Relating to the esophagus, the tubelike portion of the digestive tract between the mouth and the stomach.

exacerbation   An increase in the severity of a disease or symptom.

fiberoptic intubation   Insertion of a tube into a body passageway or hollow organ using a fiberoptic instrument. The fiberoptic device is long and thin and contains thin glass or plastic threads through which the physician can see the proper path for tube placement.

fibrillation   Chaotic, quivering, abnormal activity of the heart muscle, resulting in ineffective heart contractions.

film   Shorthand for x-ray film.

fistula   An abnormal channel that develops between two organs or from an organ to the body's surface.

Fleet   Trade name for a brand of laxative, usually referring to an enema, used to treat constipation.

forensic pathologist   A physician who specializes in examining dead bodies (when death may not have occurred naturally) and collects evidence that may be pertinent for legal investigation.

formalin   A solution used as a preservative for tissues and organs.

furosemide   A drug that increases production and excretion of urine. Commonly used to treat congestive heart failure and **edema**.

gangrene   Death of body tissue, usually due to decreased blood supply.

gastrectomy   Surgical removal of all or part of the stomach.

gastritis   Inflammation of the stomach lining.

gastrointestinal   Relating to the stomach and the intestines.

gentamicin   A type of antibiotic.

get her bloods off   Jargon for sending a patient's blood sample to a laboratory for tests.

GI   Abbreviation for **gastrointestinal**.

Glasgow Coma Scale   A system to assess response to stimuli in a person with impaired brain function, most commonly used to treat persons with head trauma.

GP   Abbreviation for general practitioner. A physician whose practice includes a wide variety of patients and medical problems.

gram-positive cocci   A group of bacteria, identified by a staining technique, that can cause various infections, such as skin and respiratory tract infections.

grand rounds   A featured educational lecture given by an expert or specialist, usually to groups of physicians, resident physicians, and medical students.

gross anatomy   The study of the structures of the body that can be seen without use of a microscope.

guaiac   A substance used in a diagnostic blood test.

gurney   A stretcher with legs on wheels that is used to transport patients.

guttate   Resembling drops.

hemolysis   The destruction or dissolving of red blood cells.

hepatosplenomegaly   Enlargement of the liver and spleen.

herpetic   Relating to or caused by the herpesvirus.

HIV   Abbreviation for human immunodeficiency virus. The virus that causes **AIDS**.

H/O   Abbreviation for history of.

Homans' sign   An indication of thrombosis (formation of a blood clot) in leg veins in which slight pain is felt in the calf muscle or at the back of the knee when the knee is bent and the foot and toes are moved upward.

hydrochlorothiazide   A drug used to treat **hypertension** and **edema**.

hydrops   Excessive accumulation of a watery fluid in body tissues or cavities.

hypercalcemia   An abnormally high level of calcium in the blood.

hyperglycemia   An abnormally high level of glucose (sugar) in the blood.

hyperimmune serum   A serum with an especially high antibody concentration.

hyperlipidemia   An abnormally high level of a type of lipid (fat) in the blood.

hyperlipoproteinemia   An abnormally high level of a type of fatty protein in the blood.

hypertension   High blood pressure.

hyperthermic perfusion   Fluid that is heated to an extremely high temperature and then infused into the patient.

hypertrophy   An increase in the thickness of tissue or size of an organ.

hypoglycemia   An abnormally low level of glucose (sugar) in the blood.

hypotension   Low blood pressure.

hypovolemic shock   Syndrome resulting from an abnormally low volume of blood in the body and characterized by **hypotension**, rapid heartbeat, and cool, clammy skin.

ibuprofen   An anti-inflammatory drug.

ICU   Abbreviation for intensive care unit.

immune adjuvants   Aids or stimulants (such as drugs) to the immune system.

immunoglobulin   Any of five different antibodies found in blood serum and tissue fluids.

induction chemotherapy   Use of drugs as the first treatment for cancer.

in extremis   At the point of death.

infarction   Shorthand for myocardial infarction (heart attack). Death of heart tissue caused by inadequate blood supply.

inotrope   Substance (usually a drug) that increases muscular contractions.

intractable   Resistant to treatment.

intubate   Insertion of a tube into the body, usually into the trachea (windpipe) to facilitate breathing.

in utero   In the uterus (before birth).

IV   Abbreviation for intravenous (ie, within a vein). Sometimes refers to the infusion of fluids into a vein.

juvenile rheumatoid arthritis   A chronic disease of the joints in children. Symptoms include inflammation, swelling, and pain.

lability   Emotional instability.

lacrimal glands   Tear ducts.

laminectomy   Surgical removal of part of a vertebra in the spine.

laparotomy   A diagnostic operation in which the abdomen is opened.

Lasix   Trade name for the drug **furosemide**.

lobectomy   Surgical removal of a lobe (part of an organ), such as from the lung or liver.

LP   Abbreviation for lumbar puncture. A diagnostic procedure in which a thin, hollow needle is inserted through the skin of the lower back and into the lower part of the spinal canal to withdraw fluid.

lumen   The cavity of a tubular organ.

lupus   Usually refers to systemic lupus erythematosus, an inflammatory disease that is characterized by fatigue, weakness, joint pain, arthritis, and skin lesions.

lymphadenopathy   Swollen lymph nodes.

lymphoma   Cancerous disease affecting the lymph system.

macular degeneration   A disorder usually occurring in older persons in which the central part of the retina of the eye deteriorates because of disease or hemorrhage; usually causes partial loss of vision but can lead to blindness.

malignancy   Usually refers to cancer that has the ability to invade and damage local tissues and to spread to other tissues or organs.

manometrics   Instruments used to measure the pressure of liquids and gases in the blood.

mastectomy   Surgical removal of all or part of a breast.

mastoid   A bone behind the ear.

medial canthus   The corner of the eye closest to the nose.

melanoma   A type of skin cancer.

meningitis   Inflammation of the membranes that surround the brain and spinal cord, usually caused by bacterial or viral infection. Symptoms usually include a stiff neck, vomiting, fever, and headache.

meningococcemia   A severe infection characterized by the presence of the bacterium **meningococcus** in the blood.

meningococcus   A bacterium that can cause **meningitis** and other infections.

metastatic   Spreading from one part of the body to another; usually refers to the spread of cancer from a primary site to a distant site.

methadone   A drug used as a substitute for heroin in the treatment of heroin addiction.

microanatomy   The microscopic study of the structure and function of cells, tissues, and organs.

micturition   Urination.

moribund   Dying.

MRI   Abbreviation for magnetic resonance imaging. A diagnostic technique that uses magnetic fields and radio waves to produce images of internal organs and tissues.

MS   Abbreviation for multiple sclerosis. A chronic disorder of unknown cause characterized by progressive degeneration of the nervous system. Symptoms may include weakness, incoordination, tingling, and speech and vision disturbances. The disease has a tendency to wax and wane.

muscular dystrophy   A degenerative disease characterized by progressive weakness and muscle wasting.

myalgias   Muscle pains.

Mycobacterium avium-intracellulare   A slow-growing bacterium that most commonly causes lung disease. Persons with **AIDS** are particularly susceptible.

myelomeningocele   A birth defect characterized by the protrusion of the spinal cord and its membranes through an abnormal opening in the spine. Also known as spina bifida.

Narc you   Jargon for the administration of narcotic drugs.

nasogastric tube   Tube inserted through the nose into the stomach. Used to drain the stomach or to administer liquids directly into the stomach to the very ill who are unable to eat.

nasotracheal intubation   Passage of a tube through the nose and into the trachea (windpipe) to facilitate breathing.

necrosis   Death of cells or tissues through injury or disease.

neuroanatomy   The branch of anatomy that deals with the nervous system.

neuroendocrine   Relating to the nervous system and the hormone system.

neurogenic bladder   Abnormal bladder function due to an impaired nerve supply.

neuropathology   A disease or abnormality of the nervous system.

neutropenic fever   Fever accompanied by the presence of an abnormally low number of a type of white blood cell.

NG tube   Abbreviation for **nasogastric tube**.

no code   Jargon for **DNR**.

nodular sclerosing Hodgkin tumors   Tumors associated with a type of Hodgkin disease (a cancerous disease affecting the lymph nodes).

oat cells   Type of cells involved in a kind of lung cancer.

occiput anterior   A position of the head of the fetus during birth with the back of the head positioned toward the front of the mother's pelvis.

odontoid process   An upward bony projection from the second vertebra of the neck around which the first vertebra rotates.

oncologist   A physician who specializes in treating patients with cancer.

OR   Abbreviation for operating room.

orchiectomy   Surgical removal of one or both testicles.

oropharyngeal Relating to the mouth and throat.

ostomy Surgical construction of an artificial opening in the abdominal wall to an organ (usually the bowel) to allow the discharge of urine or stool.

otoscope Instrument for inspecting the ear canal and eardrum.

palliation Giving relief, but not a cure; treating symptoms. Usually associated with the care of persons at the end of life.

pallor Paleness.

pancytopenia Deficiency or reduction of all cellular elements of the blood.

pannus A membrane of tissue covering a normal surface.

Pap Shorthand for Papanicolaou test. A diagnostic test in which cells are scraped from a woman's cervix and examined under a microscope to detect abnormalities. Used to screen for cervical cancer.

papilledema **Edema** of the optic disk in the eye; usually indicates increased pressure within the brain.

papule A solid, superficial elevation of the skin of less than 1 centimeter (a little less than half an inch).

parenteral Administering drugs by injection, usually intravenously or intramuscularly.

parietal bones The bones that form the sides and top of the skull.

patent Unobstructed.

pathologist A physician who specializes in the study and determination of causes of disease and death and examines tissues and organs (from living or dead persons) to establish the cause of illness or death.

pathophysiology The study of the effects of disease on body functions.

path report Shorthand for pathology report.

pauciarticular Involving only a few joints.

Peds Jargon for pediatrics. The branch of medicine that deals with the development, care, and treatment of babies, children, and adolescents.

PEEP Abbreviation for positive end-expiratory pressure. Technique used as part of mechanical ventilation consisting of administration of increased airway pressure to patients with severe lung disease to help keep air passages open and improve breathing.

Pentasa Trade name for an anti-inflammatory drug.

perfusion Flow of a liquid (such as blood) through an organ or tissue.

pericardium   The membrane that encloses the heart.

PGY-1   Abbreviation for postgraduate year 1. Clinical training after graduation from medical school. Referred to as the first year of internship or residency.

pharmacology   The science that deals with the origin, nature, chemistry, effects, and uses of drugs.

pharmacopoeia   An authoritative book on drugs and their uses. Also, a collection or stock of drugs.

pharyngitis   Inflammation of the throat.

phlebotomy   Procedure in which a vein is punctured with a thin needle (or, less often, cut with a scalpel) to remove blood.

physiology   The study of living organisms and their function.

PICU   Abbreviation for pediatric intensive care unit.

placebo   A chemically inactive substance given in place of an active drug. Used most often in the controlled experiments (known as randomized trials) that test the efficacy of the active drug. In these trials, the recipient is unaware if the substance he or she is receiving is active or inactive.

plaque   A solid, superficial, flat skin lesion often 1 centimeter (a little less than half an inch) or more in size.

Pneumocystis carinii   An organism that can cause a serious, life-threatening lung infection in persons with weakened immune systems, such as those with **AIDS**.

pneumonia   Inflammation of the lungs, most commonly due to infection with bacteria or viruses.

pneumothoraces   Plural of pneumothorax. A pneumothorax is a collection of air in the space between the chest wall and the lung that results from trauma or disease involving the chest and causes collapse of all or part of the lung.

polys   Shorthand for the white blood cells known as polymorphonuclear leukocytes.

port   A valve usually attached to an intravenous line through which medications can be injected.

preceptor   A physician who supervises and teaches a medical student.

precordial   The surface of the front of the lower part of the chest, just in front of the heart.

prednisone   A steroid drug related to cortisone, which has many actions, including anti-inflammatory effects.

pronounce her   Jargon for pronounce her dead. To officially verify that a person is dead.

prostate   Prostate gland. The organ in men surrounding the beginning of the urethra (tube leading from the bladder to the penis) that contributes to the production of semen.

prostate-specific antigen   A substance secreted in the **prostate**. Measurement of levels of this **antigen** is used as a screening test for prostate cancer.

PSA   Abbreviation for **prostate-specific antigen**.

psoriasis   A chronic skin disease characterized by circumscribed red patches covered with white scales.

PT/PTT   Abbreviations for prothrombin time/partial thromboplastin time. Tests used to determine the state of blood coagulation (clotting).

pulmonary   Relating to or affecting the lungs.

pump-oxygenator   A mechanical device that can substitute for the heart and lungs during open-heart surgery.

quadriplegic   Having paralysis of the arms and legs.

Questran   Trade name for a drug used to treat itching associated with some **gastrointestinal** diseases.

R3   Abbreviation for the third year of residency

radiography   The making of film records (radiographs) of internal structures by the passage of x-rays through the body to specially sensitized film.

radiology   The branch of medicine concerned with the diagnosis and treatment of diseases using radioactive substances (eg, x-rays).

radiolucent   Not opaque. Characterized by allowing passage of x-rays and other radiation.

rales   A rattling sound coming from the lungs and often indicating an abnormal condition.

rectal prolapse   Protrusion of part or all layers of the rectum through the anus.

Rehab   Shorthand for rehabilitation.

Relafen   Trade name for an anti-inflammatory drug.

REM sleep   Abbreviation for rapid eye movement sleep. A sleep phase during which the eye muscles contract rapidly and dreaming occurs.

Rendu-Osler-Weber syndrome   An inherited disease that usually begins after puberty. Symptoms include bleeding of the small blood vessels and capillaries into the skin and mucous membranes. Also known as hereditary hemorrhagic telangiectasia.

resection   Surgical removal of tissue or bone or of all or part of an organ.

reticuloendotheliosis   Proliferation of the cells lining the reticuloendothelial system (involving the liver, spleen, and bone marrow).

Rh   Shorthand for Rh factor. A blood group related to the presence of a certain **antigen** in blood cells. A person can have blood that is either Rh positive or Rh negative.

Rh hemolytic disease   **Erythroblastosis fetalis**.

rounds   A series of regularly scheduled visits with and assessments of hospitalized patients.

Scan you   Jargon for the examination of all or part of the body with a diagnostic scanning machine, such as a **CT scan**.

scrubs   Clothing worn by medical personnel during surgery.

Scut Monkey Handbook   Nickname for *Clinician's Pocket Reference*, a pocket-sized reference book carried and used by medical students and residents in the hospital. It contains a comprehensive compilation of diagnosis, treatment, and many other aspects of day-to-day patient care.

seizing   Jargon for having seizures.

sequelae   Conditions or outcomes resulting from disease or its treatment.

sphygmomanometer   Instrument used to measure blood pressure.

spider angiomas   Small spider-like networks of blood vessels near the surface of the skin, usually associated with pregnancy or liver disease.

spinal   Shorthand for spinal tap. A diagnostic procedure in which a thin, hollow needle is inserted through the skin of the lower back and into the lower part of the spine to withdraw fluid from the spinal cord.

stat   Immediately.

ST elevation   Elevation of a portion of an **ECG** tracing, usually indicating inadequate blood flow to a portion of the heart muscle.

sternum   The breastbone.

streptococcal   Relating to a disease-causing bacterium known as streptococcus.

streptokinase   A drug used to dissolve blood clots.

ST segment   The portion of a line on an **ECG** tracing reflecting the electrical activity of the heart.

subclavian   Located just below the clavicle (collarbone). The large vein and artery located below the clavicle are the subclavian vein and subclavian artery.

suffusions   Reddened patches on the skin resulting from injury.

symptomatology   The combined symptoms of a disease.

synaptic pathways   The site of junction between nerve cells.

syncope   Brief loss of consciousness resulting from insufficient blood flow to the brain; fainting.

systolic   Shorthand for systolic blood pressure. Blood pressure measurements include two numbers: a systolic number (the first number) and a diastolic number (the second number), eg, 120/80.

tachycardia   Rapid heartbeat.

tachypnea   Rapid breathing.

thoracentesis   Insertion of a hollow needle through the chest wall and into the space between the two membranes that cover the lungs and line the chest cavity. Thoracentesis is used to withdraw fluid.

thoracic   Relating to the chest.

thrombi   Clots formed in the heart or in a blood vessel.

thrush   Infection of the mouth caused by a yeast known as *Candida*. It occurs most commonly in persons with impaired immune function such as with **AIDS** or cancer.

toxoplasmosis   An infection caused by a protozoan parasite known as *Toxoplasma gondii*. It is generally harmless in healthy persons but could be life-threatening in persons with weakened immune systems.

tracheitis   Inflammation of the lining of the trachea (windpipe), usually caused by infection.

tracheostomy   Surgical construction of an opening through the skin and into the trachea (windpipe) to allow breathing.

urologist   A physician who specializes in the diagnosis and treatment of disorders of the genitourinary tract.

Vacutainer   Trade name for a device used to collect blood samples.

Valium   Trade name for the drug **diazepam**.

venipuncture   Puncturing a vein with a needle, usually to withdraw blood.

vent   Jargon for the treatment of a person with a **ventilator**.

ventilator   A device that helps a person breathe.

ventral   Relating to the front part of the abdomen.

V-fib   Shorthand for ventricular fibrillation. Very rapid, irregular, uncoordinated contractions of the muscle fibers in the heart.

vitals   Shorthand for vital signs. Measurement of a person's pulse rate, respiratory (breathing) rate, blood pressure, and temperature.

VP shunt   Abbreviation for ventriculoperitoneal shunt. The creation of a channel between a ventricle in the brain and the membrane that lines the abdominal wall (peritoneal cavity) using thin tubing. It is used to drain excess fluid from within or around the brain.

V-tach   Shorthand for ventricular tachycardia. An abnormally rapid heartbeat.

walking pneumonia   A mild form of pneumonia.

Washington manual   Shorthand for *Washington Manual of Medical Therapeutics*, a pocket-sized reference manual used for the management of common medical disorders.

WBC   Abbreviation for white blood cell.